FITTER
FOOD

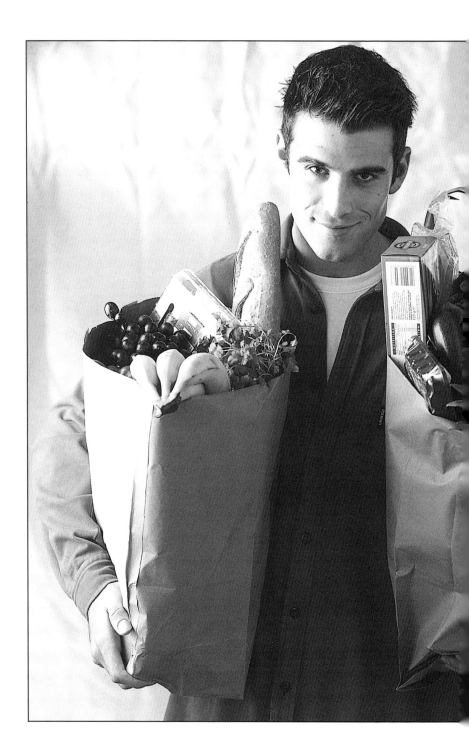

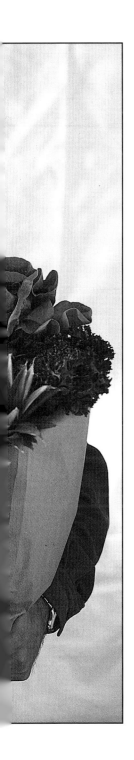

MAN ALIVE

The Ultimate Men's Guides to
Achieving Total Health

FITTER FOOD

Sarah Brewer, M.D.

MARSHALL PUBLISHING • LONDON

A Marshall Edition
Conceived, edited and designed by
Marshall Editions
170 Piccadilly
London W1V 9DD

First published in the UK in 1997 by Marshall Publishing Ltd

ISBN 1 84028 003 4

Originated in Singapore by Classicscan
Printed and bound in Portugal by Printer Portugesa

Editor	Jonathan Hilton
Art editor	Vicky Holmes
Photographer	Laura Wickenden
DTP editors	Mary Pickles, Kate Waghorn
Copy editor	Jolika Feszt
Indexer	Judy Batchelor
Managing editor	Lindsay McTeague
Production editor	Emma Dixon
Art director	Sean Keogh
Editorial director	Sophie Collins
Production	Nikki Ingram

CONTENTS

WHAT IS HEALTHY EATING?

Every man can significantly improve his life by choosing the right food.

The things a man chooses to eat are influenced by a wide variety of factors. In the West, we may learn to crave additives like salt and sugar at a very young age. Regional and cultural differences will also affect our tastes. Anyone who grew up in the north of England or Australia, for instance, is unlikely to get over the occasional craving for traditional dishes, no matter how unhealthy meat pie, chips and gravy may be. These childhood tastes are hard to kick and may stay with us for all our lives. And there is no reason why the occasional craving shouldn't be indulged. After all, delicious food is one of life's most reliable treats.

Lifestyle is also a huge influence on diet. In the modern world, many men are just too busy to settle down to cook a square meal after a hard day's work, and they may learn to depend on precooked, processed food. But with a little forethought, a healthy, satisfying and fresh meal can be thrown together in less than half an hour, which isn't much longer than it takes to wrestle your way through all the plastic packaging that comes with TV dinners.

Another factor for men making choices about what they eat is body image. Until recently, it was thought that anorexia – self-starvation – and bulimia – binging on food and then vomiting – were mainly women's disorders, but the number of men suffering from these complaints appears to be growing at an alarming

rate. A distorted body image can be extremely dangerous if it leads to unnecessary weight loss and associated muscle wastage.

A good diet means eating all the food you need to stay healthy and well-nourished. It means eating to get all the energy your body needs to carry out its continual programme of self-renewal and repair. But there's no reason why eating healthy food should be dull. Healthy food usually means tasty food, too.

The danger, especially in the West, is over-eating. For most men, getting heavier is part of getting older, but that is no reason to resign yourself to being overweight once you hit 35. Taking just a little bit of extra care with your food and exercise can mean the difference between having a beer belly and having a flat stomach.

Diets of one type or another have probably been the subject of more fads in the last 20 or so years than any other area of day-to-day living. The problem is that there is a great deal of truth in the idea that what we eat is a major contributor to our health and, by extension, to our happiness.

But diet alone, and especially dieting solely to lose weight, is never the only ingredient of good health. Regular exercise, relaxation and a sense of self-worth are all just as important. Nevertheless, if you do not eat a good, balanced diet, it is unlikely that you will be able to use your body to its full potential.

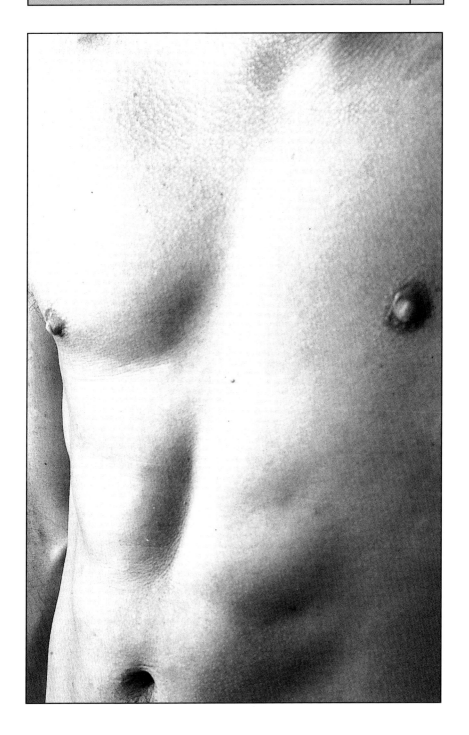

WHY EAT HEALTHILY?

As science continues to unravel the links between nutrition and health, the saying "You are what you eat" appears to have some basis in fact.

Every cell that is in your body today is made up of molecules that were not present a year ago. They have all come from one source – your food. Diet, therefore, needs to provide all the vitamins, minerals, fibre, essential fatty acids, protein and energy for good health.

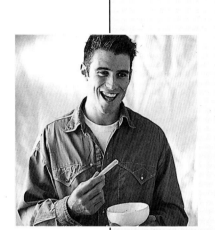

But an unbalanced diet can lead to ill health. Eating too much saturated fat, for example, may cause excessive weight gain, clogged arteries and coronary heart disease (CHD), while eating too much of certain types of polyunsaturated fatty acids and not enough of others has been linked to inflammatory diseases such as arthritis. If you eat properly, you can reduce the risk of CHD, high blood pressure (hypertension), stroke, irritable bowel syndrome, diabetes and even many types of cancer.

BODY COMPOSITION OF A YOUNG
ADULT MALE

Water	60% body weight
Protein	18% body weight
Fat	15% body weight
Minerals	6% body weight
Glycogen stores	1% body weight

◆ 2,500 kcals (*see p. 10 for definition*) energy stored as carbohydrate

◆ 12,000 kcals (80% of energy reserves) stored as fat

◆ Remaining fuel is stored as protein (such as muscle).

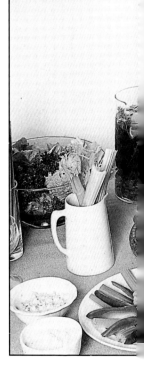

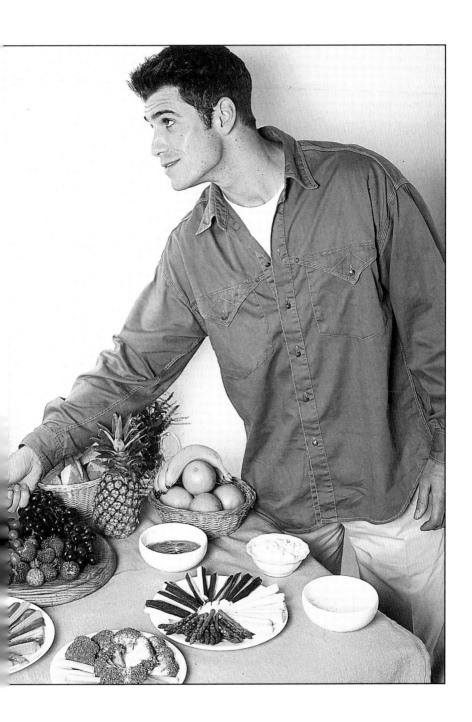

FUELLING THE BODY

Every cell in your body needs energy for growth, development and metabolic function.

The amount of energy your body needs from day to day depends on your age, your level of activity and the type of metabolism you have inherited. Most cells in your body prefer to get fuel in the form of a sugar – glucose – which is the easiest source of energy to break down.

The fuel your body depends on is measured in units known as calories. The calorie is a standard unit for measuring heat energy: 1 calorie is the amount of heat energy needed to raise the temperature of 1 gram of water by 1°C, for example, from 15°C to 16°C. This is also known as the standard calorie (cal), with a lowercase "c".

ESTIMATED DAILY ENERGY NEEDS

AGE	KCAL/DAY
11–14	2,220
15–18	2,755
19–59	2,550
60–74	2,355
75 & over	2,100

CALORIES

The unit commonly used in nutrition is the kilocalorie, or kcal. This is also known as the Calorie, spelled with a capital "C" (*compare with above*).

◆ 1 kcal = 1,000 cal

◆ 1 kg (2.2 lb) of body fat is equivalent to 7,000 kcal of stored energy.

Food provides different amounts of energy depending on its chemical structure. The body harnesses the energy stored in the chemical bonds holding the food molecules together:

◆ carbohydrates provide 4 kcal energy per gram

◆ protein provides 4 kcal energy per gram

◆ fat is the most energy-rich food available, producing 9 kcal energy per gram.

ENERGY DISTRIBUTION

Weight for weight, your brain cells require a larger supply of glucose energy than any other tissue in your body – as soon as blood sugar levels fall, both your mental function and your ability to concentrate rapidly decrease. If the blood sugar level falls too far, you may even faint. Apart from brain cells, most of the cells in your body can burn fatty acids as a source of energy, and so they are less dependent on blood sugar levels.

Muscles have the next biggest need for energy, and they are packed with energy stored in the form of a starchy substance, glycogen. Muscle cells also contain the highest concentration of the energy-processing units known as mitochondria (*see next page*).

Resting muscle cells prefer to use fatty acid molecules as their fuel

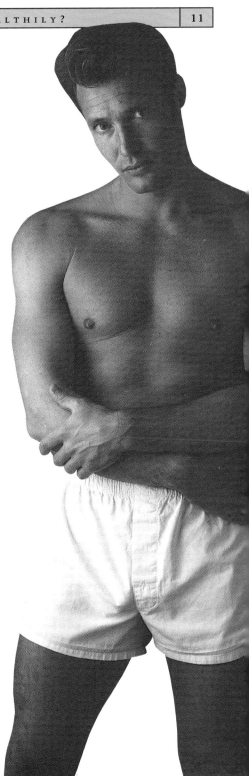

source. During exercise, their increased energy needs are met by breaking down the glycogen stored in the muscle itself and by increasing the amount of glucose taken up from the blood supply.

After a period of exercise, muscle glycogen stores are quickly replenished from the carbohydrates in your diet. If these are in short supply, your body will instead break down protein in order to regenerate the glycogen it needs.

Unfortunately, the body lacks the enzymes needed to convert fat into glucose. By eating just a small amount of glucose after exercising, you can protect your lean tissue from being broken down as an emergency fuel. This is known as the protein-sparing effect of glucose.

MITOCHONDRIA

The structures in your cells that process molecules to free the energy that their chemical bonds contain are known as mitochondria. These units have their own DNA and are the cellular equivalent of rechargeable batteries. They break down the bonds in nutrients such as glucose to form ATP, which is the body's main energy source (*see pp. 12–13*).

From a fitness point of view, regular exercise can increase both the number and the size of mitochondria within muscle cells. So your muscle cells can produce more energy and thus raise your metabolic rate (*see pp. 12–13*).

WHAT IS METABOLISM?

Your body changes food into the energy you need.

The term metabolism literally means change. It describes all the chemical and energy transformations that occur in your body, including those that convert the food you eat into energy.

Ultimately, all the elements essential for your metabolism are derived from food. This is digested and absorbed in a complex process that generates energy and stores it in small, usable parcels – chemical bonds. When these chemical bonds are broken, energy is released in a controllable way.

Most metabolic reactions depend on enzymes (complex molecules made up of protein, minerals and vitamins). These act as triggers to encourage chemical reactions that would otherwise not normally occur, or that would happen too slowly to be of much use to us.

HOW FOOD IS TRANSFORMED

During digestion, the different components present in food are broken down into smaller units: dietary proteins to amino acids; fats to fatty acids; and carbohydrates to glucose. Some are recombined to make new, complex proteins (such as enzymes),

PROTEIN MOLECULE

GLUCOSE MOLECULE

carbohydrates (such as glycogen) and fats (such as cholesterol). These are all needed for the smooth functioning of your body.

Fatty acids, glycogen and glucose do not act directly as fuel sources, however. Instead, they are used to regenerate the cells' supplies of an energy-rich molecule – ATP (adenosine triphosphate). ATP molecules store energy within their chemical bonds, and these bonds are broken down by the cells' mitochondria (*see pp. 10–11*) whenever energy is required. It is for this regeneration of ATP that oxygen, fatty acids and glucose are essential.

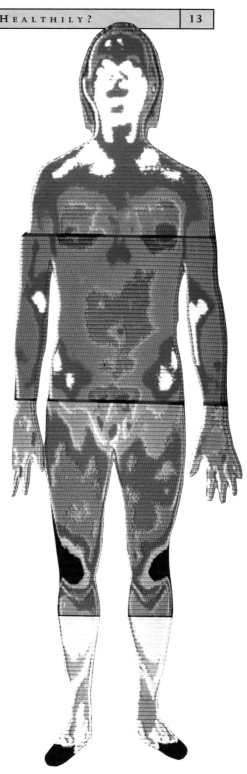

FOOD INTO ENERGY

Usually 40% of food energy is stored as chemical energy, and is used to fuel exercise and metabolism. The other 60% is given out as heat (*see heat image of a human body right – white indicates the hottest parts; purple, the coolest*). When food is in scarce supply, your metabolism becomes more efficient, and less energy is dissipated as heat.

These chemical reactions – which are known collectively as cell respiration – result in the production of both carbon dioxide and water.

FREE RADICALS

These highly reactive molecular fragments are produced as a by-product of your metabolic processes. Although they exist only momentarily, their significance lies in the fact that they carry an electrical charge which they are desperate to offload.

Free radicals do this by bombarding cellular structures, including the nucleus and genetic material, in order to "steal" an electrical charge that neutralizes their own. This can trigger a cascade of damaging reactions within the body that has been linked to such problems as premature ageing, inflammatory diseases and cancer.

Your principal protectors against metabolic free radicals are dietary antioxidants (*see pp. 16–19*), such as vitamins C and E, betacarotene and the mineral selenium. They "mop up" free radicals by neutralizing their electrical charge before they can do much harm.

METABOLIC RATE

The speed at which your metabolism operates your metabolic rate. This varies from person to person, day to day, and even hour to hour. It is partly regulated by the nervous system and partly by hormones. One's metabolic rate can be estimated by measuring the amount of oxygen used – your metabolism generates about 4.82 kcal of energy for every litre of oxygen you consume. Some of the factors affecting metabolic rates are shown in the chart below.

FACTORS AFFECTING METABOLIC RATES

	Sex	Size	Diet	Exercise
HIGH	In general, a man will have a higher metabolic rate than a woman of the same age, height and weight.	Tall people have higher metabolic rates than short people.	Food affects your metabolic rate through the so-called specific dynamic action of food. Eating 100 kcal of protein uses up 30 kcal of energy to metabolize it; 100 kcal of carbohydrate uses 6 kcal of energy; and eating 100 kcal of fat boosts metabolism by 4 kcal.	Exercise raises the metabolic rate during the period of physical activity and for a significant amount of time afterward.
LOW	Women have a lower metabolic rate partly because they have less muscle bulk in relation to their body fat.	Surprisingly, slim people have lower metabolic rates than fat people. This is because chemical reactions in fatty tissues contribute to overall metabolic rates.	Fasting and following too strict a weight loss diet slows the metabolic rate – the body responds to the threat of possible starvation by going on to red alert and improving metabolic efficiency.	Males with a sedentary lifestyle have much lower resting metabolic rates than athletes.

Emotion	Age	Health	Time of day
Stressed, anxious people have high metabolic rates due to the metabolism-boosting effect of the adrenalin hormone. They also fidget constantly, which expends so-called nervous energy.	Your metabolic rate is at its highest at age 27. After that, your metabolic rate falls each year.	Men with high levels of thyroid hormones have higher metabolic rates than those with low levels.	Your metabolic rate is highest in the morning and lowest at night.
Calm people and those suffering from the general slowing effects of a depressive illness tend to have low metabolic rates.	Between the ages of 27 and 47, your metabolic rate can fall by as much as 12%. You use up about 50 calories less per day for each five-year period after the age of 27.	Some prescription drugs (such as betablockers used to treat high blood pressure, angina, anxiety and migraine) can slow metabolic rates.	Calories eaten late at night are more likely to be converted into fat than immediately burned for energy.

DIET AND DISEASE

We are slowly coming to understand the impact on our health of what we eat.

For thousands of years, a link between diet and health had been suspected, but it was not until 1747 that a Scottish physician named James Lind proved that a specific disease was caused by a dietary deficiency. That disease was scurvy, and it was due to a lack of vitamin C.

YOU ARE WHAT YOU EAT

The saying "Let food be your medicine, and medicine be your food" illustrates how vital diet is. Most metabolic enzymes need vitamins, minerals or dietary co-enzymes to function well. If an essential micronutrient is lacking, vital regeneration and repair processes will slow down. For example:

◆ Vitamin C or zinc deficiency causes poor wound healing and easy bruising.
◆ Vitamin A deficiency causes scaly skin and inflamed gums.
◆ Vitamin B_1 deficiency causes nerve damage.
◆ Vitamin B_2, B_3, B_6, B_{12}, C, folic acid or iron deficiency causes mouth ulcers, a sore tongue and cracked lips.
◆ Vitamin B_3 or selenium deficiency causes premature wrinkles.

New research takes the health question back to your mother's diet at the time you were conceived. A poor nutrient intake during your first few weeks as an embryo might affect the way your blood vessels and organs develop, increasing your risk of high blood pressure, coronary heart disease or diabetes in later life.

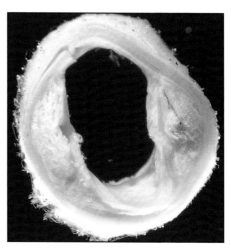

WITHOUT ANTIOXIDANTS, free radicals can attack LDL cholesterol. This is then taken up by scavenger cells, which can become trapped in artery walls to become part of the hardening and furring process.

CHOLESTEROL AND CORONARY HEART DISEASE (CHD)

It is not your total blood cholesterol level that is important, but the ratio of two types of circulating cholesterol.

◆ Low-density lipoprotein (LDL) cholesterol is linked to the hardening and furring up of arteries, high blood pressure and CHD.
◆ High-density lipoprotein (HDL) cholesterol protects against arterial disease and CHD by using up LDL cholesterol for metabolism.

Research shows that as your HDL cholesterol level rises by 1 percent, your risk of CHD falls by 2 percent. Other research has led some experts to the conclusion that eating more antioxidants – such as vitamins

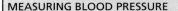

C and E, betacarotene and the mineral selenium (*see pp. 42–49*) – may protect against arterial disease, high blood pressure and stroke by preventing free radicals from attacking circulating LDL cholesterol (*see caption, previous page*).

HIGH BLOOD PRESSURE

One of the main causes of high blood pressure is the hardening and narrowing of the arteries. This occurs naturally with age, but smoking and carrying excess weight speed up the process. Other lifestyle factors that can raise your blood pressure include drinking too much alcohol, eating too much salt, stress or lack of exercise. High blood pressure runs in some families.

Because it can creep up on you without warning, high blood pressure is known as the silent killer. Even if your blood pressure is dangerously

---

MEASURING BLOOD PRESSURE

When your blood pressure (BP) is measured, as shown below, two readings are taken:

◆ The higher reading is the pressure in the system as the heart contracts and pushes blood into your circulation.

◆ The lower reading is the pressure in the system when your heart rests between beats.

These two pressures are measured against a column of mercury to see what height of mercury they can support (mmHg). The average healthy young adult man has a BP of around 120/80 mmHg at rest. But BP naturally tends to rise with age, and so a healthy, 50-year-old male may have a BP of around 150/90 mmHg. If your BP is consistently higher than 160/95 mmHg, then you are suffering from high blood pressure (hypertension).

---

high, you may feel relatively well. But some people with high blood pressure do feel dizzy or tired or suffer from pounding headaches. High blood pressure can lead to:

◆ a stroke, in which blood vessels in the brain are damaged

◆ angina (heart pain) or a heart attack, when your coronary arteries are damaged

◆ cardiac failure, in which your heart finds it difficult to pump blood around your circulatory system. This causes breathlessness, as fluids build up in your lungs

◆ failing sight, when blood vessels in the eyes are affected

◆ kidney failure, in which the blood vessels in your kidneys become damaged.

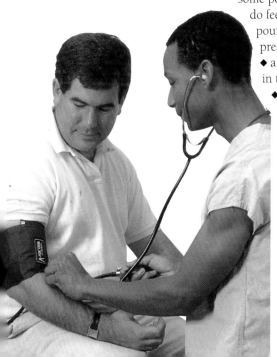

DIET AND PROSTATE CANCER

American men are 26 times more likely to develop symptoms of prostate cancer than Chinese men, and 10 times more likely to die from it than Japanese men. This is despite the fact that the numbers of men diagnosed as having early prostate cancer are approximately the same in all three countries. In China and Japan, the disease does not seem to progress. Something stops it in its tracks before it can have a fatal effect. The key to this difference is diet.

DIETARY FACTORS

It is now thought that the Eastern way of eating may be the factor that provides this protection. The traditional Japanese diet, for example, is low in fat – especially saturated fat – and consists of rice, soybeans and soybean products (such as soymeal

> ## A MODERN PLAGUE
>
> Prostate cancer is the second most common malignancy diagnosed in men in the United States:
>
> ◆ 1 out of every 11 white males and 1 out of every 10 black males will be diagnosed as having prostate cancer.
>
> ◆ American black males have the world's highest death rate from prostate cancer.
>
> ◆ More than 122,000 new cases are diagnosed every year.
>
> ◆ 20% of cases affect men under the age of 65.
>
> ◆ 30,000 men die each year from prostate cancer.

and tofu), fish (sushi), and a variety of legumes, grains and cruciferous plants (members of the cabbage and turnip families, which include kohlrabi, Chinese leaves and broccoli).

Soybeans and cruciferous plants are a rich source of weak plant hormones known as phytoestrogens. These plant hormones are released into the gut during digestion, and Japanese men have been recorded as having blood levels of phytoestrogens up to 110 times higher than men following a more Western-style of eating. These

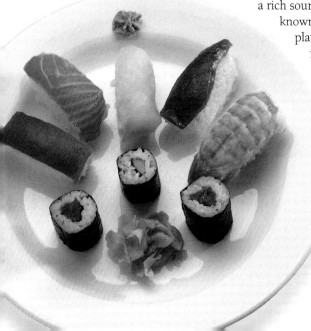

SUSHI, a traditional Japanese way of preparing raw fish, is now popular in the West. This style of eating may contribute to a healthier and longer life.

LIFESTYLE CHANGES FOR A HEALTHY HEART

FACTOR MODIFIED	REDUCTION IN RISK OF CHD
Stopping smoking	50–70% lower risk within five years of stopping
Taking exercise	45% lower risk for those who exercise regularly
Losing excess weight	35–55% lower risk for those who maintain a healthy weight
Keeping alcohol intake within healthy limits	25–45% lower risk for those drinking small to moderate amounts of alcohol
Reducing blood cholesterol levels	2–3% lower risk for each 1% reduction in cholesterol

products seem to offer some protection for the prostate gland from the effects of the male hormone testosterone and from its break-down product dihydrotestosterone, both of which have been linked to the enlargement of the prostate.

Eastern men also eat more yellow, orange, red and green vegetables than Western males. These vegetables contain antioxidants that protect against free radical attack (see pp. 12–13) and lower the risk of prostate cancer.

Research also suggests that the more fat a man eats, the higher his risk of developing symptomatic prostate cancer. Saturated fat from red meat, mayonnaise and creamy salad dressings seems to be most dangerous. Red meat has the strongest positive link, while there appears to be no increased risk from other dairy products, such as milk or cheese.

The researchers went as far as to recommend that men should take steps to lower their intake of red meat if they want to reduce their risk of developing prostate cancer. In contrast, because of their anti-inflammatory effects, essential fatty acids from nuts and seeds, omega-3 fats from oily fish and a high vitamin E diet seem to offer some protection against prostate problems.

In addition to being careful about what you eat, you may also need to change other lifestyle factors that affect your health. For example, in the case of coronary heart disease (CHD), research shows that your risk can be modified in a number of ways, as is summarized in the chart above.

THE IMMUNE SYSTEM

A nutritious diet is your first line of defence.

Your immune system is continuously fighting invaders. An army of white blood cells wages constant battle with the hundreds of germs, allergens and irritants you encounter every day. And like every standing army, your immune system needs constant supplies and a clear supply line.

IMMUNE CELLS

Your body has a number of defences against infection, including the skin and enzymes secreted in fluids such as tears and stomach juices. There are also specialized cells designed to protect against disease by attacking bacteria, viruses and foreign proteins that enter the body.

These immune cells patrol your entire body, but they are concentrated within the lymphatic system. It is this

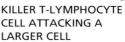

KILLER T-LYMPHOCYTE CELL ATTACKING A LARGER CELL
Three small, rounded, killer T-cells, a type of white blood cell, are seen at right. One of these smaller cells (centre) has attached itself to a large, undifferentiated cell (at right) and is attacking it. The smaller cell recognizes the cell – which may be a virus-infected cell or a cancer cell – by its surface antigens. Once it attaches itself to the larger cell, it will kill the cell, and so it acts as an important mechanism in the body's immune response to foreign bodies.

B- LYMPHOCYTES
You can see from this image of a B-lymphocyte blood cell that its surface is covered with ridges and projections, which help it to bind on to the surface of target proteins. On encountering a foreign antigen, the B-cell either divides into a number of plasma cells, which produce antibodies that kill the invader, or it matures into a memory cell. Memory cells remain in the body for years, giving immunity to the original pathogen.

system that drains and filters your tissue fluids.

When immune cells detect an infection or abnormality, they secrete chemical alarm signals known as cytokines. These signals quickly attract patrolling immune cells into an area to make a swift immune response. The main types of immune cells are shown on these pages.

All cells in your body carry surface identity "tags" that identify them as being part of you and so are not attacked by your immune system. However, a cell that is behaving abnormally through disease or infection leaves telltale chemical markers on its surface. Once these are recognized by circulating immune cells, an immediate immune response is triggered.

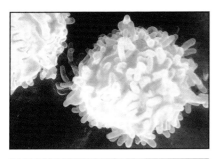

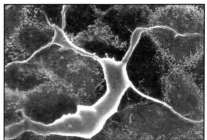

NEUTROPHILS
This type of immune cell makes up about 60% of circulating white blood cells. They engulf any invading microorganisms to halt their spread.

MACROPHAGES
These are the body's vital scavenger cells. Their job is to hunt down, then engulf, unwanted tissue debris and foreign materials.

ANTIBODIES

Antibodies, or immunoglobulins, are soluble molecules made from sugar and protein (glycoproteins). They are produced by B-lymphocytes and are present in all of your body fluids.

When an antibody encounters a foreign cell, one of your own infected body cells, or a foreign protein, its specialized shape allows it to clamp on to the particular foreign surface marker (antigen) it is designed to recognize. The antibody tail sticks out to interact with any passing immune cells, which then help to destroy the antigen-antibody complex.

DIET AND IMMUNITY

Immune cells need vitamins and minerals to carry out their tasks. Studies involving elderly people found that those taking multivitamins for a year increased their number of natural killer cells, produced a better immune response following an influenza vaccination, and suffered from infections for half as many days as those not taking supplements. Research also shows that taking supplements of vitamin C halves the risk of developing cold symptoms after exposure to the cold virus and can help symptoms to disappear more quickly.

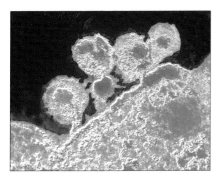

HIV AND AIDS
The human immunodeficiency virus (HIV) causes acquired immune deficiency syndrome (AIDS). T-lymphocytes that help other immune cells carry out their functions (T-helper cells) are attacked, and their numbers fall. This lowers immunity so that sufferers can be infected by organisms that do not usually harm people with a healthy immune system.

FOOD ALLERGY AND INTOLERANCE

Idiosyncratic reactions to some foods are quite common, but some can be fatal.

Several types of food intolerance and allergy can trigger adverse reactions to a general class of food or to a specific ingredient. These reactions will occur even when the food is eaten in a disguised form. For example, coeliacs have an allergy to a particular small protein found in several common cereal products, including wheat, rye, barley and oats.

In rare cases, such as severe anaphylactic reaction (*see chart below*), the body's response can be acute enough to kill the victim if professional medical treatment is not given immediately.

CHRONIC AILMENTS

Some researchers believe that lesser degrees of food allergy are also linked to such common, long-term problems as chronic fatigue syndrome, asthma, eczema, arthritis and even the hardening and narrowing of the arteries (*see pp. 16–19*).

This area of research is still controversial, but the theory is that when food is eaten, it is broken down in the intestines into its small, chemical-component "building blocks" before being absorbed by the gut. In some cases, it is thought that foods to which your immune system is

WHAT TO LOOK FOR AND WHAT TO DO

	Severe anaphylactic reaction	Gluten intolerance
CAUSE	Eating of peanuts and other related foods	Hypersensitivity to gliadin, a small protein found in gluten. Gliadin may have a direct toxic effect on the body, or it may be a victim of an over-zealous immune system.
SYMPTOMS	Life-threatening symptoms include falling blood pressure, breathing difficulties and swelling of tissue	Tiredness; general feelings of ill-health; breathlessness; abdominal pain; wind; diarrhoea; vomiting; passing bulky, fatty stools that float; weight loss; mouth ulcers and sores at the corner of the mouth
PREVENTION	Take great care to avoid these foods if you are allergic to them	Avoid gluten-containing foods if you are allergic to them

sensitive make your intestinal wall porous. This is because reactive cells found in the lining of the gut (known as mast cells) burst open to attack the food using a broad-based cocktail of toxic chemicals.

The presence of these toxic chemicals is thought to set up a low-grade inflammation in the gut wall, so that cells swell up and move apart from each other, including those in the walls of the smallest blood vessels (capillaries). As a result, incompletely digested food particles fit between the gaps left and and are then free to enter your blood stream.

Once in your system, any food particles to which you are sensitive are quickly identified and attacked by specialized immune system cells (see pp. 20–21) and destroyed. If, however, you eat too many of the foods to which your system reacts, it is thought that your immune system may become overloaded. If this occurs, food particles are allowed to roam around your body, where they become partially coated by immune proteins.

Once this stage has been reached, some researchers believe that inflammatory reactions are set up that are linked with such diseases as arthritis, eczema and asthma before the food particles are filtered out in the kidneys and finally destroyed.

At present, there is no firm evidence to confirm this theory, although much research continues in the area.

Lactose intolerance	Hypersensitivity	Food sensitivity
Inability to digest lactose sugar in milk products	Eating such foods as strawberries, eggs or shellfish	Sensitivity to chemicals found in certain foods, such as chocolate, cheese or red wine
Bloating, abdominal pain and diarrhoea	Widespread itchy rash (urticaria); eczema; asthma; vomiting; abdominal pains or diarrhoea	Can trigger migraine headaches
Follow a lactose-elimination diet in which soya or low-lactose milk products are used in place of cows' milk products	Avoid these foods if you are allergic to them	Avoid these foods if you are allergic to them

HOW YOU PROCESS YOUR FOOD

Food has to be broken down into its simplest components before the body can use it.

Your digestive system essentially processes complex food by breaking it down into simple chemical compounds, which can then be absorbed into the blood stream.

The first stages of digestion take place in the mouth as enzymes in your saliva start to break the food down. Once it has been chewed and thoroughly mixed with saliva, which also acts as a lubricant, the food travels down the oesophagus and into the stomach. Once in the stomach, chemical and mechanical action break it down much further.

From here, the food passes through the various parts of the small intestine, where it is digested further and prepared for absorption into the blood stream. In the large intestine, it is broken down even more and absorbed into the blood stream. Several different

> **THE INTESTINES**
> **The small intestine is made up of the:**
> ◆ duodenum
> ◆ jejunum
> ◆ ileum
>
> **The large intestine is made up of the:**
> ◆ caecum
> ◆ appendix
> ◆ colon
> ◆ rectum

organs and glands connected to the digestive tract aid in the digestive process (*next page*).

THE INTESTINAL TRACT

A combination of mechanical and chemical disruption breaks food down as it passes through the intestinal tract:

◆ Mechanical – muscles in the stomach wall produce a churning motion that mixes food, while coordinated contractions throughout the tract push food farther down through the digestive system.

◆ Chemical – acids, alkalis and enzymes secreted by glands in the gut wall and by associated organs (the liver and the pancreas, for example) dissolve the chemical bonds within food molecules to hasten the process of digestion.

As a result, proteins are broken down into smaller polypeptide chains and then into their constituent amino acids. Fats are broken down into fatty acids, and carbohydrates into simpler sugars.

> **CONTENTS OF STOOLS**
> ◆ 75% water
> ◆ 25% solids
> **Of which:**
> ◆ about 30% = bacteria
> ◆ about 15% = inorganic material (such as calcium and phosphates)
> ◆ about 5% = fats
> ◆ a varying percentage, depending on diet, is undigested plant fibre (roughage)
> ◆ a small amount of dead bowel-lining cells, mucus and digestive enzymes is also present.
>
> Every gram of fibre you eat adds around 5 g (about ⅙ oz) of weight to your bowel motions.

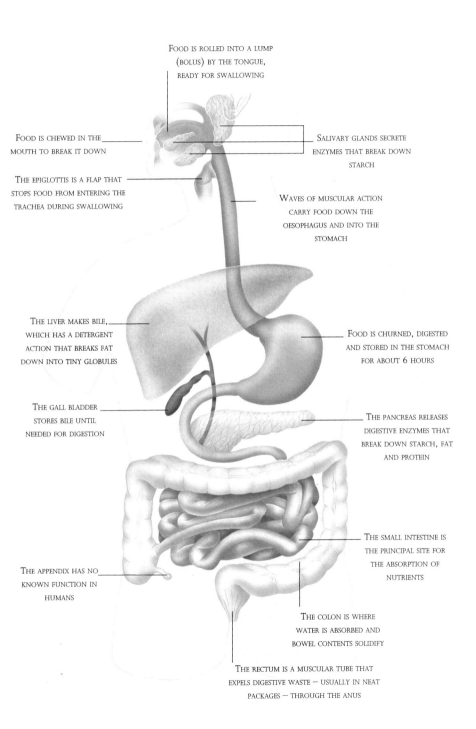

FOOD IS ROLLED INTO A LUMP (BOLUS) BY THE TONGUE, READY FOR SWALLOWING

FOOD IS CHEWED IN THE MOUTH TO BREAK IT DOWN

SALIVARY GLANDS SECRETE ENZYMES THAT BREAK DOWN STARCH

THE EPIGLOTTIS IS A FLAP THAT STOPS FOOD FROM ENTERING THE TRACHEA DURING SWALLOWING

WAVES OF MUSCULAR ACTION CARRY FOOD DOWN THE OESOPHAGUS AND INTO THE STOMACH

THE LIVER MAKES BILE, WHICH HAS A DETERGENT ACTION THAT BREAKS FAT DOWN INTO TINY GLOBULES

FOOD IS CHURNED, DIGESTED AND STORED IN THE STOMACH FOR ABOUT 6 HOURS

THE GALL BLADDER STORES BILE UNTIL NEEDED FOR DIGESTION

THE PANCREAS RELEASES DIGESTIVE ENZYMES THAT BREAK DOWN STARCH, FAT AND PROTEIN

THE SMALL INTESTINE IS THE PRINCIPAL SITE FOR THE ABSORPTION OF NUTRIENTS

THE APPENDIX HAS NO KNOWN FUNCTION IN HUMANS

THE COLON IS WHERE WATER IS ABSORBED AND BOWEL CONTENTS SOLIDIFY

THE RECTUM IS A MUSCULAR TUBE THAT EXPELS DIGESTIVE WASTE – USUALLY IN NEAT PACKAGES – THROUGH THE ANUS

WHAT IS A BALANCED DIET?

A combination of carbohydrates, protein, fat, vitamins and minerals that provides you with just the right amount of energy, with no waste, is the ideal to aim for when you are trying to devise a balanced diet.

Without a detailed professional evaluation of what you eat and the type of life you lead, you may feel that you cannot hope to know what a balanced diet actually is. The answer is to equip yourself with a few basic facts and then let common sense be your guide. A well-balanced diet should provide you with:

◆ enough energy to sustain your level of physical activity and to maintain a healthy weight

◆ enough protein for tissue repair, regeneration and rejuvenation

◆ enough essential fatty acids

◆ at least the recommended daily amount of vitamins and minerals

◆ enough fluid to maintain a normal water balance.

Different men require different amounts of nutrients, depending on their level of physical activity (both work and leisure activity), height, weight, age and rate of metabolism. Men in general obtain more than enough protein from their diets; by cutting back on fatty foods and those that are protein rich, they can make room for more of the fruit, vegetables and carbohydrates required for a balanced diet.

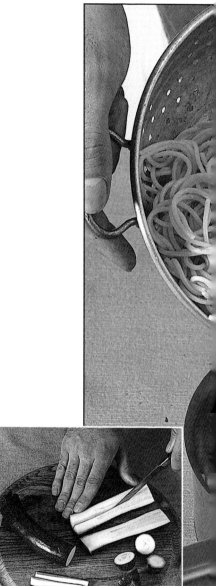

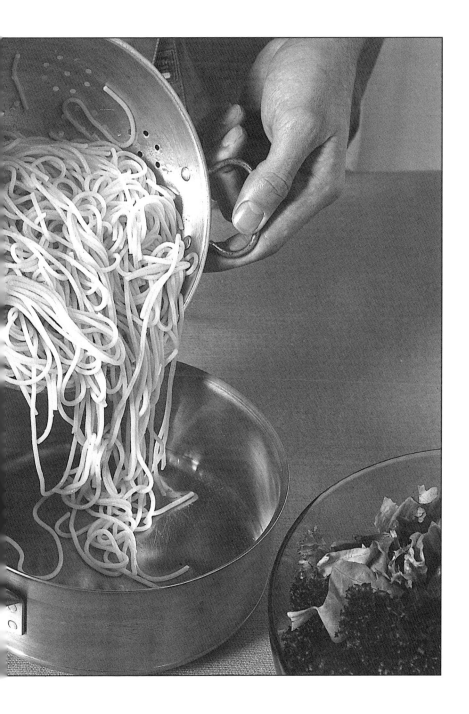

HEALTHY EATING GUIDE

Even in balanced diets, occasional treats can be allowed.

Healthy eating consists mainly of two things: establishing a balanced diet and making sure that you eat nothing in excess. You should still be able to indulge yourself occasionally, though. Use these pointers as a rough guide to a good diet, and you should find, without too much effort, that you are eating fit.

◆ Eat at least five servings of fruit and vegetables per day.

◆ Obtain 50–70 percent of your daily energy in the form of unrefined complex carbohydrates (*pp. 30–31*).

◆ Fats (*pp. 38–41*) should make up no more than 30 percent of your daily calories (around 75 g or 2½ oz for men).

◆ Saturated fats should make up no more than 10 percent of daily calories.

◆ Polyunsaturated fats should make up 3–7 percent of daily calories.

◆ Salt intake should be limited to a maximum of 6 g (⅕ oz) per day.

◆ No more than 10 percent of your daily calories should come from eating refined sugars.

◆ Eat at least 300 g (10½ oz) of fish per week.

FOOD PYRAMID

One of the easiest ways to understand healthy eating is by looking at a food pyramid. At its base are the complex carbohydrates, of which you need to eat about 5–11 servings daily. Next is the fruit and vegetable group, of which you should consume 5–9 servings per day. Animal and dairy products should each be limited to 2–3 servings daily, while at the top of the pyramid are the fats, oils, sugars and sweets which you should eat only as infrequent treats.

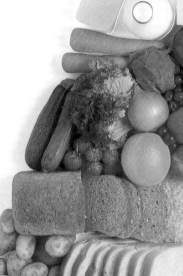

FATS AND OILS
Use very
sparingly

**MILK, YOGURT
AND CHEESE**
2–3 servings
daily

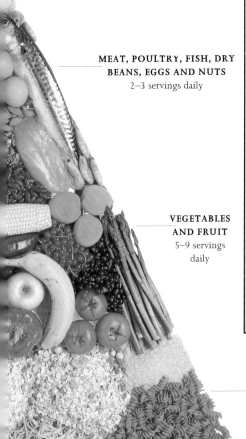

ADDED SUGAR, SWEETS,
SUGARED DRINKS
Consume infrequently

MEAT, POULTRY, FISH, DRY
BEANS, EGGS AND NUTS
2–3 servings daily

VEGETABLES
AND FRUIT
5–9 servings
daily

BREAD, CEREAL
AND POTATOES
5–11 servings
daily

WHAT IS A "SERVING"?

◆ BREAD/CEREAL/POTATO GROUP
slice of bread/toast; 3 tbsp breakfast
cereal; ½ bread bun/roll; 1 tbsp
cooked rice/pasta/noodles; 100 g
(3½ oz) boiled potatoes (2 egg-sized
potatoes).

◆ VEGETABLE/FRUIT GROUP
2 tbsp vegetables; small salad; piece
of fresh fruit; 2 tbsp cooked/tinned
fruit; 100 ml (3½ fl oz) fruit juice.

◆ MILK AND DAIRY GROUP
240 ml (½) pint milk; small pot
yogurt; 40 g (1½ oz) cheese.

◆ MEAT AND MEAT ALTERNATIVES
GROUP
55–85 g (2–3 oz) lean meat/skinless
poultry/oily fish; 110–140 g (4–5 oz)
white fish (not fried); 2 eggs (up to 6
per week), 300 g (10 oz) cooked
beans/lentils; 40 g (1½ oz) cheese.

◆ FATS (LIMIT THESE FOODS TO
3 SERVINGS DAILY)
1 tsp butter/margarine; 2 tsp low-fat
spread; 1 tsp oil; 1 tsp mayonnaise/
oily salad dressing.

◆ FATTY FOODS, CAKES AND
BISCUITS (LIMIT THESE FOODS TO
1–2 SERVINGS DAILY)
Fatty meat; luncheon meat; sausages;
rich sauces; fatty gravies; mayonnaise;
cream; cream cheese; ice cream;
pastries; pies; cakes; biscuits; chips;
crisps; packet snacks.

CARBOHYDRATES

Complex, unrefined carbohydrates are a vital component of a healthy diet.

Dietary carbohydrates provide you with most of your energy and should, ideally, make up at least 55–60 percent of your daily calories. As much of this amount as is possible should be in the form of complex, unrefined carbohydrates, such as those found in wholegrain cereals, brown rice, wholemeal bread and jacket potatoes, rather than in the form of simple sugars.

TYPES OF CARBOHYDRATE

Monosaccharides:
glucose (e.g. grape sugar)
galactose (e.g. milk sugar)
fructose (fruit sugar)

Disaccharides:
sucrose (e.g. table sugar)
lactose (milk sugar)
maltose (e.g. malt sugar)

Polysaccharides:
starch, glycogen, cellulose

SIMPLE VS. COMPLEX CARBOHYDRATES

Carbohydrates are molecules made up of carbon, hydrogen and oxygen atoms. The simplest carbohydrates are simple sugars (monosaccharides), of which the most important is glucose. Simple sugars may be joined together to form more complex double sugars (disaccharides). The best-known example is sucrose – ordinary table sugar – which is made up of glucose and fructose. Chains of sugars form what are known as complex carbohydrates – glycogen, for example.

Other complex carbohydrates, such as cellulose, cannot be digested by humans and so pass through the digestive tract (*see pp. 24–25*) virtually unchanged. They make up the bulk of dietary fibre, or roughage.

BROWN RICE
Contains more vitamins and fibre than polished white rice and is a dietary staple in many countries.

OATS
The perfect start to the day if taken as porridge or other breakfast food.

WHEATBRAN
A rich source of vitamins, fibre and complex carbohydrates.

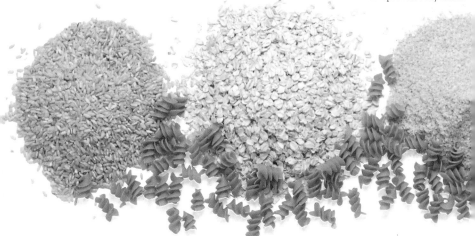

CARBOHYDRATES AND METABOLISM

Simple sugars (monosaccharides) are absorbed from the gut into your bloodstream unchanged. But before disaccharides and polysaccharides (starches) can be used by your body, they have to be broken down by the enzymes found in saliva and the gut into the simpler mono form.

Table sugar (sucrose) is easily broken down, and the resultant monosaccharides are quickly absorbed to increase blood sugar levels. Starch digestion, however, takes longer, releasing a steady stream of simpler sugars into circulation over a long period.

Unrefined complex di- and polysaccharide carbohydrates are a generally healthier nutritional option than simple sugars because they are less likely to cause large blood sugar swings and the resultant release of excess insulin. In addition, complex carbohydrates usually contain other valuable nutrients, such as vitamins, trace elements and dietary fibre. In contrast, refined carbohydrates (such as sucrose and cornflour) are highly processed, pure products consisting of pure sugar or starch, with no additional nutrients.

Once carbohydrates have been broken down into their constituent monosaccharides, they are either further processed or absorbed directly through the gut wall into the blood for distribution to the cells.

Carbohydrates trigger the release of serotonin – a brain chemical (neurotransmitter). In addition to lifting your mood, serotonin also controls the desire for food. A high-carbohydrate diet, therefore, makes you feel full quickly although you have eaten less food. You are also less likely to suffer from low moods – low serotonin levels have been linked with overeating and carbohydrate craving. Carbohydrates also boost your metabolic rate, speed up the rate at which you burn excess energy, and make you feel energized.

WHOLEMEAL PASTA
Contains more nutrients than white pasta.

BAKED POTATO
Many non-starch nutrients are lost if potatoes are peeled.

BROWN BREAD
Contains more vitamins and fibre than white bread.

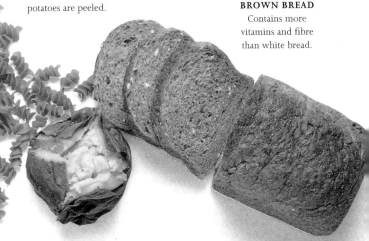

FRUIT AND VEGETABLES

Aim to eat at least five portions of fruit and vegetables every day as part of a balanced diet.

Fruit and vegetables – including nuts, seeds, pulses and wholegrains – are a rich source of nutrition. In addition to containing vitamins, protein, fibre, carbohydrates, minerals such as copper, manganese and iodine, plant hormones and essential fatty acids (*see pp. 38–41*), they are also a source of potassium, a mineral that helps flush excess sodium through the kidneys. This, in turn, reduces the risk of fluid retention and high blood pressure.

Recent research has found that plant foods contain at least 20 substances

Some nuts and seeds are rich sources of essential fatty acids that your body cannot synthesize in adequate amounts – they must, therefore, be obtained from the food you eat. However, unless you eat the 30 g (about 1 oz) of nuts or seeds per day recommended by the World Health Organization (WHO), your diet is likely to lack these vital building blocks. Evening primrose oil, in particular, is a rich source of an essential fatty acid called GLA (gamma linolenic acid). This substance acts as a building block for hormone-like

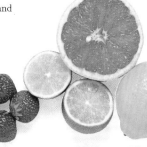

CHERRIES
A source of potassium, betacarotene and vitamin C.

STRAWBERRIES
A source of iodine, niacin and vitamin C.

CITRUS FRUITS
A source of calcium and vitamin C.

GRAPES
A source of copper, zinc, manganese and thiamin.

APRICOTS
A source of potassium, manganese, phosphorus, iron, copper, zinc and betacarotene.

that, although not nutrients, have important effects on our general health and immune system. These substances are known as phytochemicals. Many of them are plant hormones (phytoestrogens), such as a substance called genistene in broccoli that offers some protection against prostate cancer (*see pp. 18–19*).

substances known as prostaglandins. Prostaglandins are found in all tissues of the body and they play a major role in regulating inflammation, blood clotting, hormone balance and your body's immune responses against

PLANT PROTECTION

Protective dietary phytochemicals have been identified in a range of diverse foods, including green tea, olive oil and red wine, as well as in the following commonly available fruit and vegetables:

◆ apricots
◆ broccoli
◆ cherries
◆ chillies
◆ citrus fruits
◆ cranberry juice
◆ garlic
◆ grapes
◆ onions
◆ papayas
◆ parsley
◆ red peppers
◆ soy products
◆ strawberries
◆ sweet potatoes
◆ tomatoes

A much underrated food in terms of its health benefits is the walnut. This food source contains omega-3 polyunsaturated fatty acids and monounsaturated oils (*see pp. 38–41*), both of which can reduce cholesterol levels and the risk of coronary heart

ONIONS
A source of iodine, vitamin B_6, biotin and important non-nutrient antioxidants.

CHILLIES
A source of phosphorus, betacarotene, riboflavin and vitamin C.

GARLIC AND PARSLEY
Sources of antioxidants, iron, betacarotene and vitamin C.

RED PEPPERS
A source of betacarotene and vitamins E, B_6 and C.

infections and cancer. When a prostaglandin imbalance occurs (which is frequent in many men), your susceptibility to inflammatory diseases, hormonal imbalances, blood clots and skin problems such as eczema is increased.

disease. When nine healthy males added 84 g (3 oz) of walnuts to their daily diet for one month, their LDL-cholesterol levels (*see pp. 16–17*) fell by 16 percent, compared with a control group of men whose diet excluded walnuts. Increasing your intake of walnuts to just 28 g (1 oz) per day can decrease your blood LDL-cholesterol level by around 6 percent. Walnuts are also a rich source of vitamins B and E.

It is best to buy walnuts in their shells or vacuum packed, since exposure to air rapidly reduces their nutrient content.

DIETARY FIBRE

Although indigestible, dietary fibre is a vital constituent of our daily food intake.

Fibre – or roughage – provides little in the way of energy or nutrients, yet unless you have enough fibre in your diet, you will not be able to digest your food properly.

A high-fibre diet helps to prevent constipation, diverticular disease, some bowel tumours and irritable bowel syndrome. It is also thought to absorb fats, sugars, bacteria and toxins in the bowel, helping to lower blood glucose and cholesterol levels by increasing the amount of fat that is excreted.

Ideally, you need at least 30 g (1 oz) of fibre per day. An easy way to achieve this intake is to eat more unrefined complex carbohydrates, found in such foods as wholemeal bread, nuts, grains and fruits (*see pp. 30–31*).

Fibre from different plants varies widely in its composition, giving fruit and vegetables widely different textures. Think, for example, of the differences in texture between bananas and celery, tomatoes and wild rice, peas and beetroot, or asparagus and sweet corn.

SOLUBLE AND INSOLUBLE FIBRE

All plant foods contain a percentage of both soluble and insoluble fibre, although there is considerable variation in the amount each contains. In general terms, soluble fibre is completely broken down by the process of bacterial fermentation in the large intestine, while insoluble fibre is excreted.

AMOUNT OF FIBRE PER 100 g (3½ oz)	
Bran	40 g (1½ oz)
Dried apricots	18 g (more than ½ oz)
Peas	5 g (⅙ oz)
Prunes	13 g (less than ½ oz)
Brown rice	4 g (½ oz)
Brown bread	6 g (⅕ oz)
Walnuts	6 g (⅕ oz)

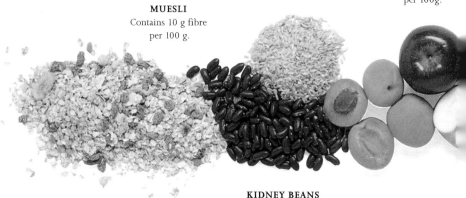

MUESLI
Contains 10 g fibre
per 100 g.

APRICOTS
Contain 18 g fibre
per 100 g.

APPLES
Contain 2 g fibre
per 100g.

KIDNEY BEANS
Contain 9 g fibre
per 100 g.

SOURCES OF SOLUBLE AND INSOLUBLE FIBRE

Type of fibre	Source	Common food examples
SOLUBLE	Oats	Porridge, muesli
	Barley	Pearl barley
	Rye	Rye bread, crispbread
	Fruit	Figs, apricots, tomatoes, apples
	Vegetables	Carrots, potatoes, courgettes
	Pulses	Cannellini beans, kidney beans
INSOLUBLE	Wheat	Wholemeal bread, cereals
	Maize	Sweetcorn, corn bread
	Rice	Brown rice
	Pasta	Wholemeal pasta, spinach pasta
	Fruit	Rhubarb, blackberries, strawberries
	Leafy vegetables	Cabbage, spinach, lettuce
	Pulses	Peas, lentils, chick peas

Soluble fibre is important in the stomach and upper intestine, where it slows digestion, ensuring that blood sugar and fat levels rise slowly, so allowing metabolism to handle nutrient fluctuations more easily.

Insoluble fibre is most important in the large intestine. It bulks up the faeces, absorbs water and hastens stool excretion. As a result, every 1 g of fibre you eat adds about 5 g (nearly ⅙ oz) to your stools. The extra weight is absorbed water and other substances – such as fat – plus the additional bulk of bacteria that multiply from the energy derived by fermenting insoluble fibre.

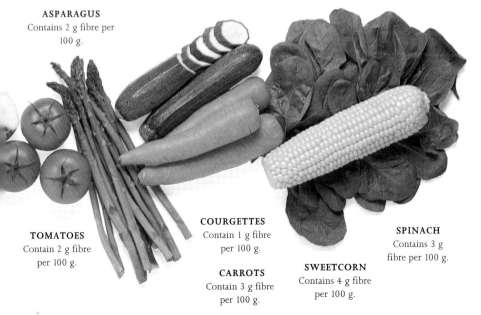

ASPARAGUS
Contains 2 g fibre per 100 g.

TOMATOES
Contain 2 g fibre per 100 g.

COURGETTES
Contain 1 g fibre per 100 g.

CARROTS
Contain 3 g fibre per 100 g.

SWEETCORN
Contains 4 g fibre per 100 g.

SPINACH
Contains 3 g fibre per 100 g.

PROTEIN

All together, more than half of the dry weight of your body is made up of protein.

Every day, about 100 g (3½ oz) of your body weight is broken down and re-formed – mostly while you are asleep – as the protein in your body is ceaselessly renewed. Most muscle protein is renewed every six months, and 98 percent of your total proteins are renewed within one year.

Proteins are made up of amino acids. These are linked together to form chains: 2–10 amino acids

RICE
Contains 3g protein per 100 g (cooked).

NUTS
Contain 18 g protein per 100 g (walnuts).

BEANS
Contain 8 g protein per 100 g (cooked kidney beans).

linked together are known as peptides; 10–100 amino acids tend to be called polypeptides; and chains of more than 100 amino acids fold into three-dimensional shapes called proteins.

Proteins in your diet are digested to release their amino acids. This process starts in the stomach, where an enzyme, pepsin, divides the linkages between certain amino acids. Once in your small intestine, these are further attacked by enzymes released from the intestinal wall and pancreas.

Twenty amino acids are important for human health. Of these, 10 cannot be synthesized in the body in amounts needed for metabolism and must, therefore, come from what you eat. Many people are surprised to learn that fruit and vegetables are a valuable source of protein, supplying about 10 percent of our daily requirements.

Protein metabolism produces a poisonous by-product, ammonia. This waste is converted into urea in the liver and is excreted via the kidneys.

CLASSES OF PROTEIN
Protein can be divided into two groups: first- and second-class proteins. First-class proteins contain significant quantities of all the essential

BROCCOLI
Contains 4 g protein per 100 g.

amino acids (those we obtain only from our diet) and are commonly found in meat, fish, eggs and dairy products.

Second-class proteins contain some essential amino acids, but not all.

SOURCES OF PROTEIN IN THE AVERAGE WESTERN DIET

◆ Meat products	36%
◆ Cereal products (mainly bread and pasta)	23%
◆ Milk and milk products	17%
◆ Fruit and vegetables	10%
◆ Fish	6%
◆ Eggs	4%

Good sources of second-class proteins are vegetables, rice, beans and nuts.

For a balanced diet, second-class proteins need to be mixed and matched by eating as wide a variety of foods as possible – for example, the essential amino acid missing from

by eating a combination of five parts rice to one part beans.

DAILY REQUIREMENTS

The average adult man needs around 56 g (2 oz) of protein per day from his food, although those taking part in competitive sports will need more (see pp. 68–71). To increase your protein intake, it is best to eat more fish, white

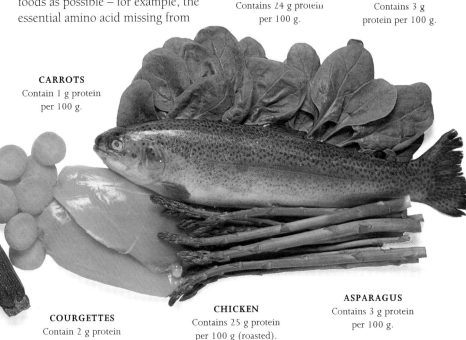

TROUT
Contains 24 g protein per 100 g.

SPINACH
Contains 3 g protein per 100 g.

CARROTS
Contain 1 g protein per 100 g.

COURGETTES
Contain 2 g protein per 100 g.

CHICKEN
Contains 25 g protein per 100 g (roasted).

ASPARAGUS
Contains 3 g protein per 100 g.

haricot beans can be found in bread. Hence, combining cereals with pulses or seeds and nuts provides a balanced intake of amino acids. Vegetarians can also obtain a balanced protein intake

meat, wholegrains, nuts, seeds and beans rather than increase your intake of some red meats and full-fat dairy products, which are also high in saturated fat (see pp. 38–41).

DIETARY FATS

Although some types of fat are known to be harmful, others can be beneficial.

Many partially understood facts about the role of fat in our diet have led people to the view that the more we can cut out, the better. However, dietary fats should provide between 25 and 30 percent of our daily energy requirements. Eating the right amounts of the right types of fat is crucial for:

♦ some essential fatty acids (*see p. 40*)
♦ cell building
♦ fatty acids necessary for the central nervous system
♦ making hormones and important hormone-like chemicals
♦ fat-soluble vitamins A, D and E.

Fats provide more than 40 percent of daily calories in the Western diet, about 16 percent of which come from saturated fat – far too high. Rather than being in the form of frying or spreading fats, which are easy to avoid, much saturated fat is hidden away in meat, cheese, milk, cakes and cookies.

WHAT MAKES FATS DIFFERENT?

When looking at the structure of fats, they all have a similar arrangement – a molecule of glycerol to which three fatty acid chains are attached. The length of these fatty acid chains and the way their atoms are bonded together dictate how the fat is metabolized in your body. In brief, the molecular variations that make fats different from each other are that:

♦ Saturated fats contain no double bonds.
♦ Unsaturated fats contain some double bonds (thus, monounsaturated fats contain only one double bond, and polyunsaturated fats two or more).

Most dietary fats are made up of varying proportions of these three types. In general, saturated fats are solid at room temperature, while mono- and polyunsaturated fats tend to be liquid.

DIETARY SOURCES

Most saturated fats come from animals (this is also the type of fat your body preferentially stores in fatty tissues). Coconut is one of the few plant sources of saturated fat. Foods rich in monounsaturates include olive oil,

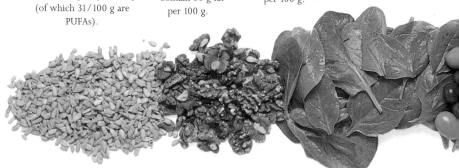

SUNFLOWER SEEDS
Contain 48 g fat per 100 g (of which 31/100 g are PUFAs).

NUTS
Contain 50 g fat per 100 g.

SPINACH
Contains 1 g fat per 100 g.

OLIVES
Contain 11 g fat per 100 g (50% monounsaturated).

rapeseed oil and avocados. These are beneficial since you metabolize dietary monounsaturated fats in such a way that they lower blood levels of harmful LDL-cholesterol (*see pp. 16–19*).

Unlike saturated fats, polyunsaturates, or to give them their full name, polyunsaturated fatty acids, or PUFAs, have spare double bonds that make them susceptible to chemical change through free radical attack (*see p. 13*). When this occurs, toxins linked with the hardening and furring up of artery walls and cancer are produced.

Factors that encourage the formation of these toxins include:
◆ eating excessive amounts of PUFAs
◆ a lack of dietary antioxidants
◆ overheating of PUFA oils so that they smoke while cooking
◆ re-using oils.

However, to understand the dietary importance of polyunsaturates, they need to be looked at more closely.

PUFAs are of two main types:
◆ omega-3 – derived mainly from fish oils – which are beneficial to health
◆ omega-6 – derived mainly from vegetable oils – which are harmful if eaten in excess.

Omega-3 fish oils have a thinning effect on the blood, reducing the risk of coronary heart disease and stroke. They also contain an essential fatty acid, derived from the algae eaten by fish, that has such beneficial effects that guidelines recommend you eat at least 300 g (10½ oz) of oily fish per week.

Fish oils have been shown to reduce the risk of rheumatoid arthritis, psoriasis, heart attack, stroke and inflammatory bowel disease.

The ratio of omega-6 to omega-3 fats in the Western diet is about 7:1, which is now thought to be too high. Omega-6 PUFAs have been linked to an increased risk of chronic inflammatory diseases, autoimmune diseases and certain types of tumours.

AVOCADOS
Contain 20 g fat per 100 g (12/100 g monounsaturated and 4/100 g saturated).

COCONUTS
Contain 68 g fat per 100 g (59/100 g saturated).

MACKEREL
Contains 16 g fat per 100 g (8/100 g monounsaturated).

VEGETABLE OILS
100% fat, made up of saturated, mono- and polyunsaturated fat.

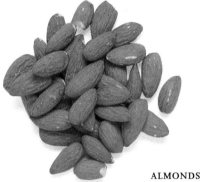

ALMONDS
A good source of linoleic acid.

ESSENTIAL FATTY ACIDS

Essential fatty acids (EFAs) are important because they act as building blocks for hormones and hormonelike chemicals known as prostaglandins. A lack of EFAs in the body has been linked with a wide range of conditions, from dry, itchy or inflamed skin, to such hormone-related problems as acne, prostate disorders and low sex drive.

The essential fatty acids cannot be synthesized in your body, and so they must come from your food. There are two EFAs:
◆ linoleic acid – an omega-6 PUFA
◆ linolenic acid – an omega-3 PUFA.

In addition, arachidonic acid – an omega-6 PUFA – may be essential if supplies in the body of other essential fatty acids (from which it can be synthesized) are low.

EFAs are found in such common foods as nuts, seeds, green leafy vegetables, oily fish and wholegrains. You can also boost your EFA levels by taking supplements, such as evening primrose oil (*see pp. 50–53*), which is a rich source of linolenic acid.

> **DIETARY SOURCES OF ESSENTIAL FATTY ACIDS**
> ◆ Linoleic acid alone is found in sunflower seeds, almonds, corn, sesame seeds, safflower oil and extra virgin olive oil.
> ◆ Linolenic acid is found in evening primrose oil, pumpkin seeds, borage seed oil and blackcurrant seed oil.
> ◆ Both linoleic and linolenic acids are found in vast quantities in walnuts, soybeans, linseed oil, rapeseed oil and flax oil.
> ◆ Arachidonic acid is found in many foods – seafood, meat, dairy products – and it can also be made from linoleic or linolenic acids.

PUMPKIN SEEDS
A good source of linolenic acid.

Scientists have found that evening primrose oil can be useful in treating such problems as irritable bowel syndrome, rheumatoid arthritis, eczema, psoriasis, high cholesterol levels and high blood pressure.

It is estimated that as many as 8 out of 10 men do not get enough EFAs from their diet. What is more, the metabolic pathways in the body that are involved in the processing of EFAs can become blocked by excessive consumption of saturated fat, sugar and alcohol; a lack of vitamins and minerals, and by smoking cigarettes or being excessively stressed.

TRANS-FATTY ACIDS

When polyunsaturated oils are partially hydrogenated to solidify them in the production of cooking fats and spreads, such as margarine, chemical substances known as trans-fatty acids are produced. When these are incorporated into your cell membranes, they increase their rigidity. Trans-fatty acids also seem to raise blood levels of LDL-cholesterol and lower HDL-cholesterol levels (*see pp. 16–19*). These substances have, therefore, been linked to an increased risk of coronary heart disease. They may also interfere with the way your body handles essential fatty acids so that their beneficial effects are not fully realized.

SUNFLOWER SEEDS
A good source of linoleic acid.

content. In Denmark, for example, new guidelines aim to reduce intakes of trans-fatty acids from margarine from 5 g per day to no more than 2 g per day.

Small amounts of trans-fatty acids are also found in milk, cheese, butter and meat, but these naturally occurring trans-fats are structurally different from those produced commercially during hydrogenation of fats, and they have, so far, not been implicated in increasing coronary heart disease risk.

This has turned the butter vs. margarine controversy on its head – now some scientists believe that it is healthier to eat butter than margarine or low-fat spreads. The simplest advice is to eat as wide a variety of foods as possible, including a little of everything (such as butter and margarine) and nothing to excess.

SESAME SEEDS
A good source of linoleic acid.

The average consumption of dietary trans-fatty acids is 5–7 g (about ¼ oz) per day. But if you use cheap margarines and lots of processed foods you could be consuming 30 g (1 oz) daily. Concern about their safety is great enough that some margarines and low-fat spreads are being reformulated to reduce their trans-fat

WALNUTS
A good source of both linoleic and linolenic acid.

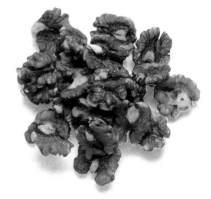

VITAMINS

Needed only in minute amounts, vitamins are, nonetheless, crucial.

These naturally occurring organic substances either cannot be synthesized in the body at all, or are made only in amounts that are too small to meet your needs (for example, vitamin D and niacin). Vitamins must, therefore, come from your food.

Most vitamins act as essential intermediaries or catalysts to keep your metabolic reactions running smoothly and efficiently. These reactions include:

◆ converting fats and carbohydrates into energy
◆ digestion of foods
◆ cell division and growth
◆ repair of damaged tissues
◆ healthy blood
◆ fighting infection
◆ mental alertness
◆ healthy reproduction
◆ mopping up harmful by-products of metabolism, such as free radicals.

Vitamins are classified into two main groups:

◆ The fat-soluble vitamins (A, D, E and K) dissolve in fat and are stored in the body – mainly in the liver.

◆ The water-soluble vitamins (B-group vitamins and vitamin C) are easily lost in urine. These vitamins cannot be stored in the body in any appreciable amounts (with the exception of vitamin B_{12}), and they must be continually replenished from your diet.

VITAMIN C

HOW MUCH IS NEEDED (adult males):
Around 60 mg per day.
Some evidence suggests that 500 mg per day or more may be beneficial.

WHAT IT DOES:
◆ acts as a powerful antioxidant
◆ is essential for the synthesis of collagen – a major structural protein in the body
◆ is necessary for healthy skin, bones, teeth and reproduction
◆ is a natural antihistamine
◆ has antiviral and antibacterial actions.

HARMFUL IN EXCESS?
In huge quantities, may cause indigestion or diarrhoea.

SYMPTOMS OF DEFICIENCY:
Poor wound healing; dry, scaly skin; broken thread veins in skin around hair follicles; brittle hair; scalp dryness; hair loss; dry, chapped lips; easy bruising; loose teeth; inflamed, bleeding gums; bleeding skin, eyes and nose; muscle and joint pain; irritability and depression.

GOOD FOOD SOURCES:
Blackcurrants, guavas, kiwi fruit, citrus fruit, mangoes, green peppers, strawberries, green sprouting vegetables and potatoes.

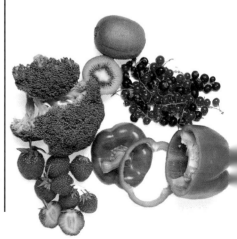

B-GROUP VITAMINS

HOW MUCH IS NEEDED (adult males):

Vitamin B_1 (thiamine)	1.4–1.5 mg per day.
Vitamin B_2 (riboflavin)	1.6–1.7 mg per day.
Vitamin B_3 (niacin)	18–19 mg per day.
Vitamin B_5 (pantothenic acid)	6 mg per day.
Vitamin B_6 (pyridoxine)	2 mg per day.
Vitamin B_{12} (cobalamin)	1–3 mcg per day.
Folic acid	200–300 mcg per day.
Biotin	100–150 mcg per day.

WHAT THEY DO:
◆ play a central role in metabolism and the way nerves and muscle cells conduct messages
◆ are essential for the production of energy from blood sugar and fatty acids
◆ are essential for the production of red blood cells, which transport oxygen
◆ are needed for healthy bone marrow
◆ are involved in the synthesis and replication of DNA
◆ are used in the synthesis of amino acids
◆ in association with chromium, niacin is essential for the interaction of insulin with its cell receptors to control glucose uptake by the body
◆ some vitamins in this group are important antioxidants.

HARMFUL IN EXCESS?
Large doses of niacin (B_3) –in excess of 30 mg per day (which is less than double the recommended daily amount) – may cause pronounced flushing and can lead to nausea, headache, muscle cramps, diarrhoea and low blood pressure. Very high doses – in excess of 2 g daily – are toxic and can cause liver damage.
Excess vitamin B_6 – more than 100 mg per day – may lead to reversible nerve damage (felt as tingling and burning sensations, shooting pains and pins and needles) and even partial paralysis in some instances.
Note: Folic acid supplements can interfere with anti-epilepsy medication.

SYMPTOMS OF DEFICIENCY:
Tiredness; pallor (anaemia); headaches; loss of appetite; nausea; constipation; irritability; loss of concentration; poor memory; difficulty in sleeping; difficulty in coping with stress; depression; blood shot, red eyes; sores and cracks at the corners of the mouth; red, inflamed tongue and lips; mouth ulcers; scaly eczema-like skin rash, especially on the face and nose; muscle weakness and general stiffness.
Note: People with a high alcohol intake are especially at risk of vitamin B_1 (thiamine) deficiency, since alcohol requires thiamine for its metabolism.

GOOD FOOD SOURCES:
Brewer's yeast and yeast extracts, brown rice, wheat germ and wheat bran, wholemeal bread and cereals, oatmeal and oatflakes, soya flour, pasta, meat and offal, milk and dairy products, seafood, green leafy vegetables, beans and nuts.
Note: Vitamin B_{12} (cobalamin) is found only in animal products, so strict vegetarians, and especially vegans, are potentially at particular risk of B_{12} deficiency, leading to anaemia.

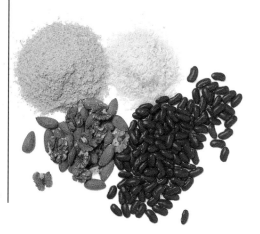

VITAMIN E

HOW MUCH IS NEEDED (adult males):
About 10 mg per day.
Some evidence suggests that intakes of
40 mcg per day or more may be
beneficial in some circumstances.

WHAT IT DOES:
◆ is a powerful antioxidant
◆ protects body fats (cell membranes,
nerve sheaths, cholesterol molecules)
from free radical attack and rancidity
◆ strengthens muscle fibres
◆ boosts immunity
◆ improves skin suppleness and healing.

HARMFUL IN EXCESS?
May cause minor gastrointestinal upsets.
Should not be taken if you are on blood-
thinning tablets unless closely monitored.

SYMPTOMS OF DEFICIENCY:
Lack of energy; lethargy; poor
concentration; irritability; lowered
sex drive; muscle weakness.

GOOD FOOD SOURCES:
Wheatgerm oil, avocados, margarine,
eggs, butter, wholemeal cereals, seeds,
nuts, bread, oily fish, broccoli.

VITAMIN A (RETINOL)

HOW MUCH IS NEEDED (adult males):
About 800 mcg per day.

WHAT IT DOES:
◆ regulates the way in which genes are
read to produce enzymes and other
proteins
◆ controls growth and development,
sexual health and reproduction
◆ maintains healthy skin, teeth, bones
and mucous membranes
◆ converts into the pigment visual purple
(rhodopsin), which is involved in sight
and night vision.

HARMFUL IN EXCESS?
Vitamin A is toxic in excess. It can cause
nausea, headaches, visual disturbances,
skin problems, coma and death. Only
four times the recommended intake may
be harmful for some men.

SYMPTOMS OF DEFICIENCY:
Increased susceptibility to infection; scaly
skin; raised, pimply hair follicles; flaking
scalp; brittle, dull hair; poor eyesight and
night vision; dry, burning, itchy eyes; eye
ulceration; kidney stones; inflamed gums
and mucous membranes.

GOOD FOOD SOURCES:
Offal, dairy products, eggs.

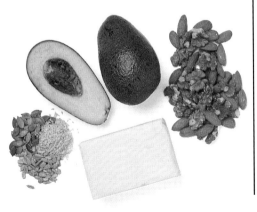

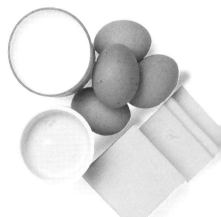

PROVITAMIN A (BETACAROTENE)

Consists of two vitamin A molecules joined together. 6 mcg betacarotene is nutritionally equivalent to 1 mcg vitamin A.

HOW MUCH IS NEEDED (adult males):
About 6 mcg per day (minimum).

WHAT IT DOES:
Same as vitamin A (*previous page*).

HARMFUL IN EXCESS?
Daily intakes above 15 mg per day may turn skin a yellow-orange colour – this is not harmful. However, high intakes by smokers have been linked to an increased risk of lung cancer. Best taken along with other antioxidants, such as vitamins E and C.

SYMPTOMS OF DEFICIENCY:
Same as vitamin A (*previous page*).

GOOD FOOD SOURCES:
Dark green leafy vegetables, such as spinach, broccoli, and parsley; carrots, sweet potatoes and yellow-orange fruits.

VITAMIN D

HOW MUCH IS NEEDED (adult males):
5–10 mcg per day.
It is naturally synthesized in your skin via exposure to sunlight.

WHAT IT DOES:
◆ acts as a hormone (calcitriol)
◆ helps absorb dietary calcium and phosphate in the small intestine.
◆ is essential for healthy bones and teeth.

HARMFUL IN EXCESS?
If taken in excess, it leads to high blood calcium levels, thirst, anorexia and kidney stones.

SYMPTOMS OF DEFICIENCY:
Constipation; muscle weakness; lowered immunity with increased susceptibility to infections; poor growth; irritability; bone pain and deformity; deafness (in osteomalacia).

GOOD FOOD SOURCES:
Oily fish – such as sardines, herring, mackerel, salmon, tuna – fish liver oils, liver, eggs, fortified milk, butter.

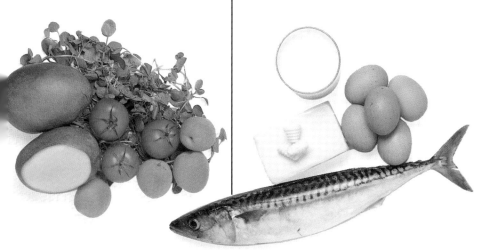

MINERALS

An average adult male contains about 3 kg (6½ lb) of minerals.

Essential for some metabolic reactions are minerals – inorganic elements, some of which are metals. Those needed in amounts of less than 100 mg per day are often referred to as trace elements. Minerals and trace elements can come only from your diet, and the quantities found in food depend on the quality of soil on which the produce was either grown or grazed.

   Most of the minerals found inside the body are in the skeleton. Minerals perform a number of functions:

◆ Calcium, magnesium and phosphate help the structure of the body – for example, strengthening bones and teeth.

◆ Sodium, potassium and calcium help to maintain normal cell function.

◆ Copper, iron, magnesium, manganese, molybdenum, selenium and zinc may be a factor in the formation of enzymes.

◆ Iron is involved in the transportation of oxygen around the body.

◆ Chromium and iodine are part of the normal functioning of hormones.

◆ Several minerals act as antioxidants (*see pp. 18–19*), the most important being selenium, manganese, copper and zinc. These protective substances patrol the body, mopping up harmful by-products of metabolism.

   Some trace elements – such as nickel, tin and vanadium – are known to be essential only in tiny amounts to regulate normal growth. However, their exact roles in the body are not yet fully understood.

CALCIUM

HOW MUCH IS NEEDED (adult males):
About 800–1,200 mg per day.

WHAT IT DOES:
◆ helps to maintain the body's structure
◆ is involved in nerve conduction, muscle contraction and energy production
◆ is needed for blood clotting, the actions of some enzymes, as well as immune functions.

HARMFUL IN EXCESS?
High intakes may be linked to an increased risk of kidney stones.

SYMPTOMS OF DEFICIENCY:
Muscle aches, pains, spasms or cramps; palpitations; receding gums; infected gums; periodontal disease; loose teeth; convulsions; dementia.

GOOD FOOD SOURCES:
Dairy products, green leafy vegetables (such as broccoli), salmon, nuts, seeds, pulses and eggs.

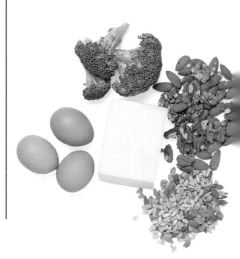

CHROMIUM

HOW MUCH iS NEEDED (adult males):
About 50–200 mg per day.

WHAT IT DOES:
Forms a complex substance known as the Glucose Tolerance Factor, which helps to control glucose metabolism.

HARMFUL IN EXCESS?
Food-grade chromium (trivalent) seems non-toxic. However, hexavalent chromium (like that found on metal car bumpers) is highly toxic.

SYMPTOMS OF DEFICIENCY:
Poor glucose tolerance with either raised or lowered blood sugar levels; poor tolerance of alcohol; abnormal blood fat levels; muscle weakness; hunger pangs and weight gain; nervousness; irritability; decreased sperm count and impaired fertility.

GOOD FOOD SOURCES:
Brewer's yeast, egg yolk, red meat, cheese, fruit and fruit juice, wholegrains, black pepper, thyme.

IODINE

HOW MUCH IS NEEDED (adult males):
About 150 mcg per day.

WHAT IT DOES:
Is needed for the production of two thyroid hormones – thyroxine and tri-iodothyronine – that control the body's metabolic rate.

HARMFUL IN EXCESS?
Decreases thyroid function, and it may also lead to dermatitis or make acne worse.

SYMPTOMS OF DEFICIENCY:
Underactive thyroid gland; swollen thyroid gland (goitre); tiredness; lack of energy; muscle weakness; susceptibility to the cold; coarse skin; brittle, coarse hair; weight gain; increased production of mucus.

GOOD FOOD SOURCES:
Marine fish (such as haddock, halibut, salmon and tuna), seafood (such as prawns, mussels, lobster and oysters), seaweed, iodized salt, milk (cattle feed is also iodized).

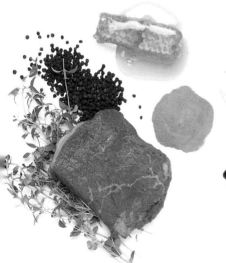
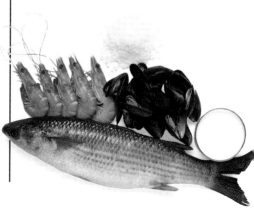

IRON

HOW MUCH IS NEEDED (adult males):
About 14 mg per day.

WHAT IT DOES:
◆ is essential for the production of haemoglobin, which transports oxygen and carbon dioxide around the body
◆ is found in a protein called myoglobin, which binds oxygen in muscle cells
◆ is involved in many reactions involving energy production and immunity.

HARMFUL IN EXCESS?
May lead to liver damage.

SYMPTOMS OF DEFICIENCY:
Pallor (anaemia); general fatigue; muscle fatigue; itchy skin; brittle nails; brittle hair and hair loss; dizziness; headaches; insomnia; sore tongue; difficulty swallowing; cracking at the corners of the mouth; decreased appetite; increased susceptibility to infection; rapid pulse; shortness of breath.

GOOD FOOD SOURCES:
Shellfish, fish, brewer's yeast, offal, red meat.

MAGNESIUM

HOW MUCH IS NEEDED (adult males):
About 300–350 mg per day.

WHAT IT DOES:
◆ maintains the electrical stability of the cells
◆ regulates the heart beat
◆ is vital for every major metabolic reaction.

HARMFUL IN EXCESS?
No evidence of toxicity as long as heart and kidneys are functioning normally.

SYMPTOMS OF DEFICIENCY:
Poor appetite; nausea; fatigue; muscle trembling; weakness; muscle cramps; numbness and tingling; loss of co-ordination; diarrhoea/constipation (early/late deficiency); insomnia; hyperactivity; low blood sugar.

GOOD FOOD SOURCES:
Soy beans, nuts, seafood, seaweed, meat, eggs, dairy products, dark green leafy vegetables.

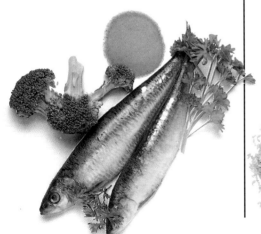

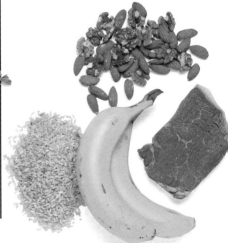

SELENIUM

HOW MUCH IS NEEDED (adult males):
About 70–75 mcg per day.

WHAT IT DOES:
◆ is essential for cell growth and immune function
◆ is involved in the synthesis of hormone-like substances, prostaglandins and antibodies
◆ acts as a powerful antioxidant.

HARMFUL IN EXCESS?
May result in hair loss, nail problems, gastrointestinal problems and nerve damage.

SYMPTOMS OF DEFICIENCY:
Hair, nail and skin problems; premature wrinkling of skin; poor growth; arthritis; impaired fertility; high blood pressure; cataracts; some cancers.

GOOD FOOD SOURCES:
Broccoli, cabbage, celery, mushrooms, onions, garlic, nuts, seafood, offal.

ZINC

HOW MUCH IS NEEDED (adult males):
About 15 mg per day.

WHAT IT DOES:
◆ is essential for the proper functioning of more than 100 enzymes
◆ is vital for growth, sexual maturity, wound healing and immune function.

HARMFUL IN EXCESS?
Can cause stomach upset and nausea.

SYMPTOMS OF DEFICIENCY:
Poor growth; delayed puberty; underdeveloped sex organs; low sperm count; impaired fertility; impotence; poor wound healing; skin problems such as eczema, psoriasis and acne; poor hair and nail growth; impaired immunity and increased risk of infection; loss of taste and smell sensations; poor appetite.

GOOD FOOD SOURCES:
Red meat and offal, seafood (especially oysters), brewer's yeast, wholegrains, pulses, eggs and cheese.

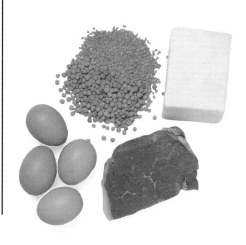

WHY TAKE SUPPLEMENTS?

Even if your diet is well balanced, you may still need to take certain supplements.

Increasing numbers of nutritional experts now believe that taking a food supplement is essential for optimal health. While your diet should always come first, taking a multinutrient supplement may be an easy and reassuring way to safeguard your future well-being.

DEFICIENCIES IN PERSPECTIVE

Minor vitamin and mineral deficiencies are surprisingly common. It is estimated that only 1 man in 10 gets all the vitamins, minerals and essential fatty acids he needs from his food. In the West, these deficiencies are rarely severe enough to result in diseases such as scurvy, but they can be bad enough to impair your immunity and increase your susceptibility to poor health. Surveys conducted in Western countries suggest that:

♦ 60 percent of the population obtains less than 60 mg vitamin C per day
♦ 90 percent obtains less than 10 mg vitamin E per day
♦ 90 percent obtains less than 2 mg betacarotene per day
♦ average intakes of both vitamins B_1 and B_2 are below recommended levels
♦ 50 percent of adults obtain less vitamin B_6 than is ideal
♦ 56 percent obtain less vitamin D than is ideal.

The situation with minerals is even worse, with large proportions of the population at risk of gross deficiency. The average man obtains only:

♦ 53 percent of the recommended intake of zinc
♦ 68 percent of the recommended intake of iron
♦ 78 percent of the recommended intake of magnesium.

If this were not bad enough, 40 percent of men obtain less dietary calcium than is recommended, and the average intake of selenium in some countries is less than 50 percent of recommended daily levels.

LIFESTYLE FACTORS

Although vitamin and mineral deficiencies are often thought of as being problems associated with women, men are just as likely to be deficient in these vital nutritional components, especially if they are physically active or lead a busy life.

♦ Athletic men, in particular, will benefit from additional B-group vitamins, which are needed to release energy in muscle cells (*see pp. 64–69*).
♦ Sexually active men are more likely to be deficient in mineral zinc than women are, since each ejaculation contains about 5 mg zinc – which is one-third of the recommended daily amount.
♦ If you smoke cigarettes, regularly drink more alcohol than is recommended as being safe, or you are under prolonged stress, your need for certain minerals and vitamins – especially the B-group vitamins and the antioxidants – increases.

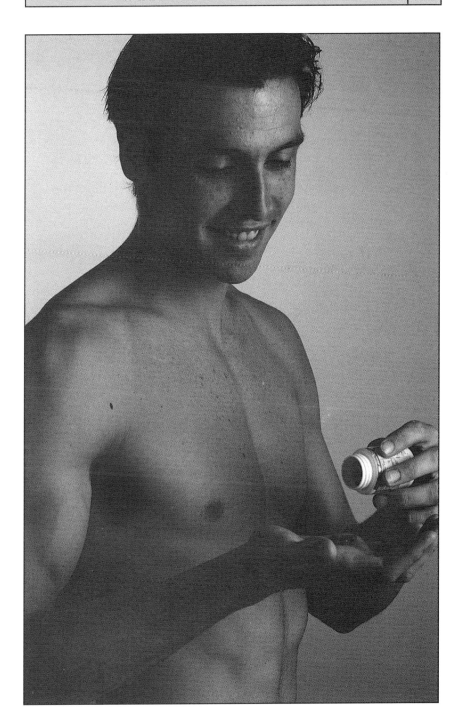

SUPPLEMENTS AND THEIR BENEFITS

Some men take supplements specifically targeted to meet their dietary requirements, while others take a more broad-based, multinutrient approach. The following overview looks at some popular supplements and the potential benefits they can bring.

MULTIVITAMINS/MINERALS
A lack of vitamins and minerals may adversely affect growth, immunity, energy production, healing, digestion, nerve function, fertility,

FISH-OIL SUPPLEMENTS
Taking omega-3 fish-oil supplements has been shown to boost immunity, to decrease the risk of blood clots and to have a beneficial effect on blood fats. They can also reduce the risk of high blood pressure, stroke and CHD, and can improve the symptoms of eczema, asthma and chronic inflammatory diseases such as arthritis.

EVENING PRIMROSE/STARFLOWER OIL
Supplements made from oil extracted from evening primrose and starflower (borage) can help a wide range of problems, including

VITAMIN C
Helps to increase the absorption of iron in the gut. It is best taken separately from inorganic selenium (but not organic selenium), since it may impair selenium absorption.

and the general maintenance of your body tissues. However, some "mega-dose" supplements can be potentially harmful, since they contain more of some nutrients than are needed by the majority of people. As a general rule, choose a supplement that has about 100 percent of the recommended daily amount (RDA) for as many vitamins and minerals as possible.

GARLIC TABLETS
Garlic powder tablets have been found to lower blood pressure by 17%, reduce the risk of stroke by up to 40%, reduce the risk of coronary heart disease (CHD) by up to 25% and improve the circulation of blood to the skin and peripheries by as much as 55%.

POPULAR FOOD SUPPLEMENTS

Of the scores of supplements available in specialist and general food stores, these are the most popular:

◆ fish oils – omega-3s and cod liver
◆ multivitamins and minerals
◆ evening primrose oil
◆ garlic capsules
◆ single vitamins and minerals – vitamins C, B-complex and E, zinc, iron and calcium
◆ antioxidants – vitamins A, C and E, betacarotene and selenium
◆ ginkgo
◆ ginseng
◆ blue-green algae
◆ royal jelly
◆ aloe vera
◆ propolis – a resinous substance gathered by bees from trees.

irritable bowel syndrome, rheumatoid arthritis, high cholesterol levels, high blood pressure, brittle nails and acne.

ANTIOXIDANTS

These supplements can help to protect against premature ageing, cataracts, hardening and furring of the arteries, CHD, stroke, chronic inflammatory diseases, and cancers of the mouth, throat, larynx, oesophagus, stomach, large intestine, bladder and lung.

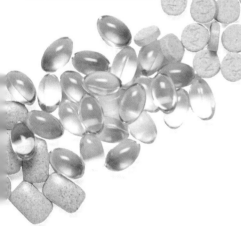

CHROMIUM

If this supplement is taken in the form of picolinate, it has been shown to help muscle cells absorb more amino acids than other versions, making it beneficial for athletes in training.

BLUE-GREEN ALGAE

Having evolved more than 3 billion years ago, blue-green algae are the world's oldest food source. They provide more vitamins, minerals and protein per acre than any other source. In addition to providing essential fatty acids and all eight amino acids (in optimum proportions), they seem to be an immune enhancer and have been found to help treat cancer, peptic ulcers and toxicity from heavy metals.

IRON SUPPLEMENTS

If you take these supplements in isolation, they may decrease the absorption of dietary zinc, manganese, chromium and selenium.

DIET AND LIFESTYLE

Lack of time, difficulty in sticking to an eating plan, or having to dine out a lot can make following a healthy diet difficult. To succeed, you need three things: an idea of your goal, a plan of action and plenty of motivation.

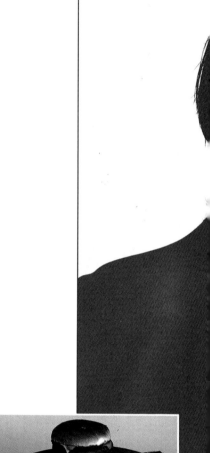

Knowing the healthy options to choose from restaurant menus, for example, or insisting on a grilled steak with fresh herbs instead of a fat-laden sauce, may be all that is needed to keep you on the right track.

Try to eat regular meals at regular times to keep your blood sugar levels even. But if a snack attack does occur, be prepared with a bag of apples, dried fruit or unsalted nuts (especially walnuts).

If you are a sportsman, you will probably already have a generally good knowledge of how to eat healthily. But you may not be aware of how much carbohydrates, water, vitamins or minerals you need. Even when you follow a healthy diet, your food may not be as nutritious as you think – poor soil, the way products are stored and processing all have an effect. Taking sensible supplements will help keep your performance at peak levels.

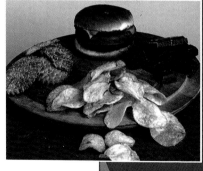

Personal advice is invaluable. If you can, take guidance from a sports nutritionist who can help you to tailor your eating regime to suit your lifestyle and level of physical training.

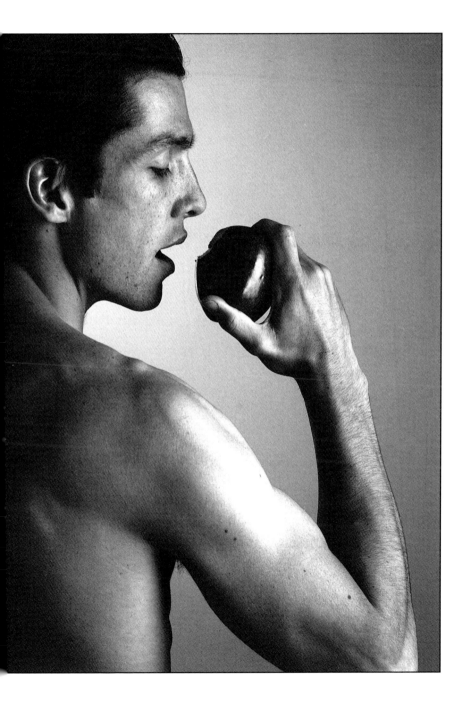

FOOD FACTS

The more you know about the food you eat, the easier it is to eat fit.

You rely on the quality of your food to obtain all the nutrients for life, but there are some basic facts you should know before you buy.

◆ Crops are frequently grown in artificially fertilized soils boosted with nitrogen, phosphorus and potassium but depleted of other minerals and trace elements.

◆ Crops are bred for good colour and shape, not for flavour and nutrients.

◆ Pesticides interfere with the · nutritional content of food plants.

◆ Foods shipped from abroad may be picked before they are ripe – nutrient content then falls with increasing age.

◆ Additives used in processing can interfere with nutrients.

◆ Produce rapidly loses vitamins after harvesting – even after a few days.

◆ Cooking decreases the level of nutrients of food plants even further.

FRESH VS. CANNED AND FROZEN

In an ideal situation, you could shop every day for fresh, organically grown food that has received minimum processing and contains maximum goodness. For most of us,

however, the reality is different. Organically grown food is expensive (weight for weight, but not in nutrient content per weight) and difficult to find in any great variety. And time constraints mean that you may be able to shop only once a week for most of your food requirements.

But there are steps you can take to get the best that is available.

◆ Look at the label and, whenever possible, buy only seasonal foods grown in your own country. Most food stores indicate the country of origin of their produce.

◆ If foods are not labelled, ask for more information before buying.

◆ Buy organically grown food whenever it is available.

In terms of taste, texture and, especially, nutrient content, fresh fruit and vegetables are definitely superior to either canned or frozen, but since fresh produce is not always available, here are some basic facts:

TV DINNERS
Although the ingredients of TV dinners may seem nourishing, these highly processed, prepared food items are likely to be severely deficient in essential nutrients.

◆ Canning vegetables destroys 20–35 percent of their vitamin A content, up to 80 percent of their vitamin E and 20 percent of their vitamin B_6.

◆ Thawing and cooking frozen vegetables removes 40 percent of their vitamin B_6 content.

◆ Frozen foods can lose up to 70 percent of their vitamin E content within 14 days of processing.

◆ Fruit and vegetables can lose more than 50 percent of their magnesium content when frozen.

◆ Once fruit juice is opened, its vitamin C content rapidly falls. Virtually all is lost within 14 days.

◆ Freezing meats reduces riboflavin by up to 50 percent.

◆ Vitamin B_5 content of food is slowly destroyed by freezing.

EFFECTS OF PROCESSING

◆ Curing meat reduces its vitamin B_{12} content by up to 40 percent.

◆ Processing wheat can reduce its vitamin B_5 content by 60 percent.

◆ Up to 90 percent of folate in grain is lost during milling.

◆ Cereals and grains lose more than 90 percent of their vitamin E content during processing (in the production of white flour).

◆ Grains lose 80 percent of their magnesium during milling.

◆ Chopping or mincing allows up to 70 percent of a food's thiamin content to be lost into cooking juices – this is reclaimable if the juices are consumed.

FISH

Fresh fish should smell of sea water – salty and slightly sweet – but not of fish. Before buying fish, keep a lookout for:

◆ eyes that are clear, bright and shiny
◆ firm skin
◆ tight scales
◆ gills that are a healthy pink or bright red

TAKE-AWAY MEALS
Even the best-quality ingredients suffer from being cooked in advance and then reheated before finally being eaten.

◆ flesh that springs back when prodded
◆ shellfish (lobsters, crabs, mussels, scallops, oysters, etc) that seem heavy for their size
◆ molluscs – those with two shells, such as mussels and oysters – that shut firmly when they are tapped.

MAKING THE MOST OF YOUR FOOD AND DRINK

By cooking your food in the healthiest way possible, the fat content of your diet can be minimized and the nutrient content optimized. Preferred methods of cooking include steaming, grilling (with only a light brushing of olive or rapeseed oil, plus herbs, lemon juice and spices), dry baking, boiling (with only the minimal amount of water and no added salt), dry (stir) frying using a brushing of olive oil.

TIPS ON COOKING MEAT

◆ When roasting meat, place it on a rack within the roasting pan so that the fats and juices drain away.

◆ When roasting chicken, use a glass funnel roaster on which you prop the chicken vertically in the oven. All the fats will then drain off, leaving you with beautifully flavoured, low-fat meat and virtually fat-free skin.

◆ When making gravy, use the water the vegetables were cooked in to retain flavour and nutrients.

TIPS ON EATING OUT

It is when we are eating out – socially or on business – that it is most difficult to stick to a diet plan. The temptation always is to have that little food treat you would not normally be tempted by, or to eat a little

> **SAMPLE MENU (INCLUDING FIVE PORTIONS OF FRESH FRUIT AND VEGETABLES A DAY)**
> Healthy eating guidelines encourage you to eat at least five servings of fresh fruit and vegetables per day in order to obtain enough antioxidants. This may seem a lot, but is relatively easy to do:
> **BREAKFAST:** glass of orange juice with your cereal or toast.
> **MID-MORNING:** have an apple or some other piece of fruit.
> **LUNCH:** a large mixed salad to accompany your meal.
> **MID-AFTERNOON:** have a banana or some other piece of fruit.
> **EVENING:** one or two portions of vegetables as part of your meal.

DINING OUT
Study the menu carefully to find the healthiest eating options. If you do not see what you want, ask for it.

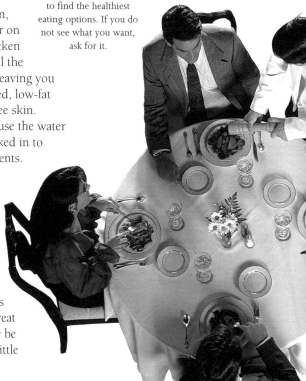

more heavily than you know is really good for you. If eating out is just an occasional activity for you, then no harm will be done by choosing all of your favourite foods. If, however, your business or social life means you are in a restaurant a few times a week – every week – then here are some tips on what to order.

◆ Pass on the bread roll and butter.

◆ Avoid deep-fried foods. Go for grilled, baked or steamed instead.

◆ Choose fish instead of red meat.

◆ Eat white meat with its skin removed.

◆ Ask for all visible fat to be trimmed from the meat before cooking.

◆ Ask to have buttery or creamy sauces left off.

◆ Do not choose anything that is wrapped in pastry, fried, battered or stuffed.

◆ Opt for Chinese, Malaysian or Japanese dishes – these are often low in hidden fat.

◆ Choose plain boiled rice rather than fried rice.

◆ Avoid pasta with rich, creamy sauces. Go for tomato, fish or clam sauces instead.

◆ Choose pizzas with plain tomato, garlic and vegetable toppings rather than meat or cheese ones.

◆ Have yogurt or fromage frais as a dressing instead of mayonnaise or cream.

◆ Choose fruit, sorbets or low-fat cheese and biscuits instead of creamy, sweet desserts.

ALCOHOL CONSUMPTION

Drinking a moderate amount of alcohol, especially red wine, may lower the risk of coronary heart disease by about 25 percent. This is mostly due to the powerful antioxidants found in red wine and the thinning effect of alcohol on the blood.

If you drink excessive amounts of alcohol, however, your risk of CHD is increased. Men who regularly drink more than six alcoholic drinks in one session are at twice the risk of sudden death than those who drink only moderately (two to four drinks a day). Try to limit your weekly alcohol intake to a maximum of 21–28 drinks spread throughout the week – aim to have several alcohol-free days, too. Tips on cutting back on alcohol include:

◆ When drinking alcohol, sip slowly. Putting your glass down rather than holding it in your hand will reduce the amount you sip by habit.

◆ Alternate each alcoholic drink with a nonalcoholic one. Nonalcoholic fruit juice cocktails can be delicious and full of nutrients.

◆ Drink mineral water with a dash of fresh lemon juice.

◆ Tonic water with ice, lemon and a dash of Angostura bitters is a great substitute for a gin and tonic.

◆ Mix chilled white or red wine with sparkling mineral water.

◆ Drink fruit/herbal teas – these are delicious, and since they are usually drunk without milk or sugar, they have the additional bonus of being calorie-free.

How many calories you need

The number of calories you need each day depends on your level of activity as well as your metabolic rate (*see pp. 12–15*). Use this chart to find out how many calories you are likely to need to maintain your body weight in respect of your age and activity level. Bear in mind that these figures are estimated averages only; some men will need more, others less.

Example 1

A 28-year-old, stressed executive who spends all day on the phone at his desk, and takes no exercise will need about 2,500 kcal if he weighs 75 kg (165 lb). He will also need to watch his alcohol intake, try not to smoke, and to limit his intake of caffeine. He will need to ensure that he gets plenty of vitamins and minerals by eating healthily and taking a good, multinutrient supplement.

Example 2

Someone the same age and weight as above who travels a lot and is averagely active will need around 3,000 kcal per day. He may also need to make healthy food choices from menus in restaurants.

Example 3

A manual worker may need 4,000 kcal per day to maintain his weight. Extra calories should come from complex carbohydrates, not sugary and fatty foods. He will also need more vitamins and minerals than the average male, and it may be worthwhile taking a good multinutrient supplement.

Pattern of physical activity

LEVEL 1: PHYSICALLY INACTIVE MALE
Spends most of his day sitting at a desk, reading, watching TV, writing, listening to the radio. Plays no sport and only rarely gets his pulse up above resting levels.

LEVEL 2: MILDLY ACTIVE MALE
Spends most of his day driving, doing general office work, pottering around the home, doing light laboratory work or playing a musical instrument. Takes occasional short walks, but these are rarely brisk.

LEVEL 3: AVERAGELY ACTIVE MALE
Spends half the day on his feet as a professional or technical worker, an administrator or manager, student, sales representative, clerical worker, teacher or lecturer. Has regular, light physical activity, such as gardening or playing sport once a week.

LEVEL 4: ACTIVE MALE
Spends a lot of time on his feet as a sales or service worker, painter, roofer, window cleaner, carpenter, joiner, motor mechanic. Physically active in leisure time, taking part in cycling or sport at least twice per week and is used to pushing himself.

LEVEL 5: VERY ACTIVE MALE
Has a strenuous job as an equipment operator, labourer, agricultural worker, forestry worker, fisherman, bricklayer, mason, construction worker or builder, or plays physically active sports at least three times a week.

ESTIMATED ENERGY REQUIREMENTS FOR ADULT MALES (KCAL/DAY)

19–29 years					30–59 years				
60 kg 130 lb	65 kg 145 lb	70 kg 150 lb	75 kg 165 lb	80 kg 175 lb	65 kg 145 lb	70 kg 150 lb	75 kg 165 lb	80 kg 175 lb	85 kg 190 lb
2,220	2,340	2,435	2,555	2,650	2,270	2,340	2,435	2,510	2,580
2,390	2,510	2,625	2,745	2,840	2,435	2,510	2,600	2,700	2,770
2,720	2,840	2,985	3,100	3,225	2,745	2,840	2,960	3,055	3,150
3,200	3,340	3,485	3,630	3,795	3,225	3,345	3,460	3,580	3,700
3,510	3,675	3,845	4,010	4,180	3,560	3,680	3,820	3,940	4,060

VEGETARIANS

Eating a vegetarian diet makes you five times less likely to need hospitalization.

Men who are concerned about what they eat and follow a healthy diet enjoy a lower risk of such common diseases as obesity, gallstones, diverticular disease, coronary heart disease and even cancer – especially of the lungs and colon. These beneficial effects may partly be due to other lifestyle factors – vegetarians are more likely to take regular exercise, for example, and are less likely to smoke or drink excessive amounts of alcohol.

Because meat is a valuable source of many important nutrients, vegetarians, and particularly vegans, must obtain these nutrients elsewhere in their diet. This is not difficult and, in general, vegetarians tend to have higher intakes of betacarotene, thiamin, folate, vitamin C, vitamin E and fibre than non-vegetarians. Their intake of iron, calcium and vitamin B_{12} may, however, be lower than a meat-eater's.

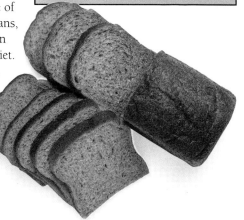

IRON

Common non-meat sources include:
- egg yolk
- brewer's yeast
- wheatgerm
- wholemeal bread
- fortified breakfast cereals
- prunes and other dried fruit
- green vegetables
- parsley
- cocoa
- curry powder

VITAMIN B_{12}

This vitamin is derived mainly from animal sources, and most vegetarians are aware of the need to watch their intake of this important nutrient. Several sources of vitamin B_{12} are suitable for vegetarians. These include:
- yeasts enriched with vitamin B_{12}
- preparations made by bacterial fermentation
- extracts derived from blue-green algae, such as spirulina, chlorella and aphanizomenon flos-aquae.

STAPLES

Bread provides an essential amino acid missing in other non-meat foods, so it is a good idea for vegetarians to eat bread on a regular basis.

TIPS FOR VEGETARIANS

The following suggestions outline the ideal content of a typical vegetarian diet. Aim to eat:
- as wide a variety of foods as possible
- wholegrain cereals rather than refined cereals
- at least 50 percent of your daily

calories in the form of complex carbohydrates, such as brown bread and wholewheat pasta
♦ three to four servings of cereal and grains per day to provide calories, protein, fibre, B vitamins, calcium and iron
♦ at least 500 g (17½ oz) fruit and vegetables per day
♦ dried fruits for fibre and iron
♦ two large portions of carrots or sweet potatoes (yams) per week for betacarotene
♦ two to three servings of pulses, nuts and seeds per day for protein, energy, fibre, calcium, iron, zinc and vitamin E
♦ nuts, seeds, pulses and cereals for protein. No single food contains all the essential amino acids, so combining cereals with pulses or seeds and nuts provides a balanced amino acid intake
♦ textured vegetable protein (TVP) made from soy beans is an excellent source of protein, calcium, iron, zinc, thiamin, riboflavin and niacin
♦ mycoprotein, which is derived from a fungus, is a good source of protein – commercially available products may contain egg white

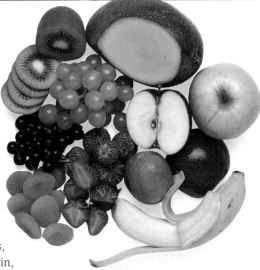

TASTE AND FIBRE
Eating as wide a variety of fruit and nuts as possible on a daily basis is one of the foundation stones of a healthy and balanced intake of fibre and nutrients for vegetarians.

♦ 475 ml (1 pint) of semi-skimmed milk (or fortified soy milk) per day for protein, calcium and trace minerals
♦ a serving of low-fat or nonfat cheese per day for protein, calcium and minerals
♦ three or four eggs per week
♦ olive and rape seed oils in cooking for important monounsaturated fats
♦ nuts, seeds and evening primrose oil for essential fatty acids.

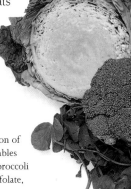

SALAD DAYS
Eat a large salad or portion of dark green, leafy vegetables (for example, spinach, broccoli or greens) per day for folate, calcium and iron.

CALCIUM
Common non-meat sources include:
♦ milk, including soy milk
♦ dairy products, such as cheese, yogurt, fromage frais
♦ green leafy vegetables
♦ salmon
♦ nuts and seeds
♦ pulses
♦ fortified cereals
♦ eggs

SPORTS NUTRITION

The more sport you play, the more nutrients you need to fuel your metabolism.

To perform at peak levels, sportsmen need to obtain more vitamins, minerals, cofactors, amino acids and essential fatty acids from their diet than sedentary men.

> **PHYSIOLOGICAL DEMANDS**
> The harder you train, the more nutrients you need to:
> ◆ maintain your red blood cells, which carry oxygen to muscles
> ◆ maintain muscle bulk and increase strength
> ◆ maintain your metabolic reactions at a high rate
> ◆ supply muscles with fuel.

The shortage of even a single nutrient may cause a metabolic imbalance that impairs your performance – lack of folic acid or iron, for example, can cause anaemia, since both are needed to make haemoglobin. It is also important to obtain the nutrients in the right balance. Too much of one vitamin may interfere with the metabolism of another. Excess zinc, for example, affects iron metabolism, while excess iron affects the way your body handles copper.

MUSCLE FUEL SOURCES

During exercise, metabolic activity and heat output within your muscle cells can increase to more than 20 times their resting rate. Resting muscles prefer to use fatty acids as fuel. However, during exercise your muscles take up glucose from the blood stream as well as breaking down their own stores of carbohydrates (glycogen). Muscle glycogen stores are expandable – a man with a sedentary lifestyle will have around 1 g of glycogen per 100 g of muscle, while a trained athlete may have as much as 4 g glycogen per 100 g.

Fat stores are of little immediate help during exercise; they have to be broken down into fatty acids before they can be used as fuel. This takes time and, during intense exercise, it is easier for muscles to burn protein as fuel if glucose is in short supply. By increasing your intake of carbohydrates, which are quickly metabolized to release glucose, you can stop the breakdown of muscle protein as an emergency energy source. Muscles with a plentiful supply of glycogen are able to exercise longer without tiring. In turn, this increases muscle bulk and increases the amount of glycogen you can store.

ANAEROBIC EXERCISE

If during strenuous exercise all stores of ATP (*see pp. 12–13*) are used up, or oxygen is in short supply, a molecule, phosphorylcreatine, comes into play. This is a rich source of energy, which, unlike the energy in ATP, can be tapped without the need for oxygen. This is known as anaerobic (without oxygen) metabolism and provides muscles with an additional "spurt" of strength in times of danger or stress.

You cannot exercise anaerobically for long, since you build up an "oxygen debt" that has to be paid back during the recovery period. Anaerobic exercise also results in a build up of lactic acid and other chemicals that cause rapid tiring and cramps. By forming an oxygen debt that you can pay back later (when gasping for breath after exertion), you are capable of six times the exertion that would otherwise have been possible.

◆ In a 100-m sprint taking 10 seconds, 85 percent of energy used comes from anaerobic metabolism, since your circulation cannot keep up with your muscles' oxygen demands.

◆ In a 3-km (2-mile) race taking 10 minutes, 20 percent of energy is produced anaerobically.

◆ In a long-distance race lasting 60 minutes, only 5 percent of energy is derived anaerobically, since your rate of exercise is slower.

After exercising anaerobically, you still need oxygen to remove lactic acid and replenish stores of ATP and phosphorylcreatine.

As you get fitter, you can increase the oxygen supply to your muscles more easily – this is why exercise leaves you feeling less breathless and tired when you have been training. You will be able to exert yourself more strenuously without a build up of lactic acid, and incur a smaller oxygen debt for a given amount of exertion as a result of:

◆ increased muscle bulk

◆ larger glycogen stores

◆ opening up and expansion of the circulation in your muscles so that blood and oxygen are brought in more quickly (pumping-up effect)

◆ developing a more efficient cardio-respiratory system.

All of these effects rely on your getting enough energy in your food, preferably as complex carbohydrates, to prevent your protein stores being used as an emergency fuel source.

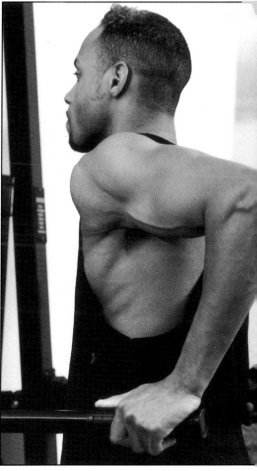

BENEFITS OF EXERCISE
Exercise builds up muscle bulk, stimulates the production of mitochondria and increases muscle glycogen stores.

FLUIDS AND ELECTROLYTES

During exercise, you lose an increased amount of body fluid as sweat, which is designed to cool you down as it evaporates from your skin. Even with constant fluid replenishment and cool surroundings, heavy exercise can increase your body temperature to as much as 39.4°C (103°F) within 15 minutes – about 37°C (98.6°F) is normal.

In addition to an increase in body temperature, sportsmen in intensive training can also lose as much as 10 litres (20 pints) of fluid per day, which needs constant replenishing. Sweat loss can be so high when running a marathon, for example, that severe dehydration may result. If your muscles are dehydrated by just 3 percent, muscle strength will fall by as much as 10 percent – your performance will literally dry up.

If you are in serious training for a long-distance endurance event, such as a marathon, you can improve your body hydration beforehand by following the advice on the right.

ELECTROLYTES

Although sweat and urine contain dissolved salts, sportsmen lose much more water than salt during intense and prolonged exercise. You need to replace this fluid loss by drinking at least a 475 ml (1 pint) of plain bottled water before you start drinking sports drinks (*right*) of electrolyte solutions or those containing glucose.

These drinks are specially designed to replace fluid loss (after the plain-water intake). They also provide an

BODY HYDRATION FOR A MARATHON

◆ Increase your intake of dietary carbohydrates for a week before the event – these are stored in your body as glycogen, which mops up water like a sponge. Each 1 g of glycogen can bind 2.7 g of water.

◆ Drink extra water during the 48 hours before the event.

◆ Starting four hours beforehand, drink 200 ml water every 15 minutes until half an hour before.

◆ Drink nothing in the final half hour to ensure that all the fluid is absorbed and that your stomach is empty.

◆ During an endurance event such as a marathon, you will also need to take fluids.

◆ Water taken before and during the event should either be plain water or contain only low quantities of sugar.

◆ Avoid fizzy drinks or those containing more than 7 percent sugar, since this will slow down absorption.

◆ You will need to empty your bladder just before the event, but once you start exercising, your urine output will fall as a result of increased secretion of anti-diuretic hormones.

◆ Since every male has a different capacity to store water, try this waterload regime several times during training to make sure it suits you.

SPORTS DRINKS

Hypotonic drinks
These are less concentrated than body fluids. They contain 2–3 g of carbohydrates per 100 ml of liquid.

Isotonic drinks
These contain the same concentration of salts as body fluids do plus 6–7 g of carbohydrates per 100 ml of liquid.

Carbohydrate or energy drinks
These contain high quantities of dissolved sugar at 10–20 g per 100 ml of liquid.

vitamins and minerals are best taken at the end of the day, when stores of some nutrients, such as calcium, are in greatest flux; most growth, repair and regeneration processes also occur at night. If you are taking supplements, it may be best to spread out your intake by taking half the dose in the morning and half in the early evening.

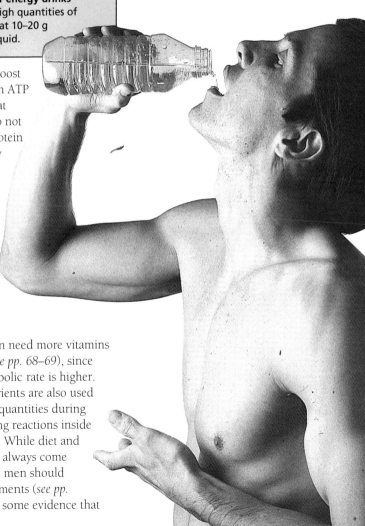

instant energy boost to help replenish ATP molecules so that your muscles do not have to burn protein as an emergency fuel source (*see pp. 64–65*). The box above gives details of the three main types of sports drinks.

VITAMIN AND MINERAL REQUIREMENTS

Active sportsmen need more vitamins and minerals (*see pp. 68–69*), since their basal metabolic rate is higher. Many other nutrients are also used up in increased quantities during energy-processing reactions inside the muscle cells. While diet and eating fit should always come first, most active men should also take supplements (*see pp. 50–53*). There is some evidence that

VITAMIN	DO SPORTSMEN NEED MORE THAN USUAL AMOUNTS?	AMOUNTS SUGGESTED BY SOME NUTRITIONISTS FOR ACTIVE SPORTSMEN
B_1	Yes	50–100 mg/day
B_2	Yes	2–2.5 mg
b_3	Yes	25–50 mg
B_5	Yes	20–100 mg
B_6	Yes	10–25 mg
B_{12}	Possibly	2–20 mcg
FOLATE	Yes	400–800 mcg
C	Yes	1–2 g
D	no	Up to 10 mcg
E	Yes	20–400 mg
MINERAL		
CALCIUM	Yes	400–1,000 mg
CHROMIUM	Yes	50–200 mg
IODINE	Yes	50–150 mcg
IRON	Yes	10–15 mg
MAGNESIUM	Yes	400–500 mg
MANGANESE	Yes	2 mg
PHOSPHORUS	Yes	1 g
POTASSIUM	Yes	100–200 mg
SELENIUM	Yes	50–200 mcg
ZINC	Yes	15–20 mg

AMOUNTS SOMETIMES ADVISED (UNDER SUPERVISION) FOR ATHLETES IN FULL TRAINING	REASON EXTRA AMOUNTS ARE NEEDED
100–200 mg/day	For the production of energy
25–200 mg	To boost oxygen consumption and performance
50–100 mg	For the production of energy
100–200 mg	To reduce production of lactic acid
25–50 mg	for the production of energy
20–50 mcg	For the production of energy and red blood cells
800–4,800 mcg	For the production of energy and red blood cells
2–12 g	To neutralize free radicals produced during exercise
Up to 10 mcg	Extra not required
400 mg–2 g	To neutralize free radicals produced during exercise
1,000–1,600 mg	For muscle contraction, nerve conduction and healthy bones
200–800 mg	For the production of energy from glucose
150–200 mcg	To replace that lost in sweat
15–25 mg	For the Production of haemoglobin
500 mg–1 g	To replace that lost in sweat
5 mg	For synthesis of amino acids and energy
1–4 g	To boost stamina and performance
200–500 mg	To replace that lost in sweat
200–400 mcg	To neutralize free radicals produced during exercise
20–50 mg	To replace that lost in sweat

BULKING UP

Some men find it as hard to put on weight as others do to lose it.

While some people seem to have an excess-weight problem (*see pp. 72–73*) a few have the opposite to contend with – being underweight. Putting on weight, or bulking up, is often recommended before an endurance competition that lasts more than two hours. Pre-loading your muscles with glycogen stores can improve your performance by boosting your stamina – in other words, you can continue at your maximum pace for longer. For shorter athletic events, glycogen loading is not usually recommended. The glycogen would tend to slow you down because you would not be exercising long enough to benefit from the extra weight (glycogen in addition to its associated water stores) you would be carrying.

To boost your muscle glycogen stores, you need to ensure that your diet contains at least 60 percent of calories in the form of carbohydrates (*see pp. 30–31*). As a rough guide, the average athlete would need to eat around 650 g (23 oz) of carbohydrates per day when glycogen loading. This will vary depending on your body weight, your chosen sport, how hard and long you train, and the way your body handles carbohydrate metabolism. Some athletes may need to double this intake of carbohydrates, while some may need to halve it – a sports nutritionist can work with you to help you determine your optimum carbohydrate intake when glycogen loading.

Glycogen loading of muscles only works if your increased carbohydrate intake is accompanied by intensive training so that your muscles are initially depleted of glycogen. Although it sounds contradictory, this process triggers glycogen synthesis and stops excess dietary carbohydrates from being converted into fat.

By depleting your muscle glycogen during training, your muscles will respond by becoming loaded with more glycogen than you started with. During training, this depletion-loading cycle is repeated several times to maximize your muscle glycogen stores before an event.

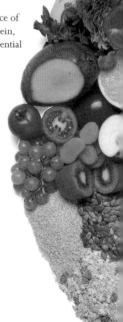

VEGETABLES
These are an excellent source of carbohydrates, fibre, protein, vitamins, minerals and essential fatty acids.

FRUIT
Using fresh fruit as healthy between-meal snacks will make a positive addition to your daily calorie intake.

Only the muscles used during exercising will deplete and load with glycogen. It will not automatically occur throughout all your muscles. You need, therefore, to make sure your gym work combines light weights with high repetitions that exercise your legs, arms, neck, shoulders and back muscles. If you attend a gym, a personal trainer can help you work out a suitable regime.

CAKES, SWEETS AND BISCUITS
Eating these types of highly refined food will soon pile on the weight, but it is likely to be in the form of flab.

TIPS FOR HEALTHY WEIGHT GAIN
If you feel that you are underweight, the following advice, combined with increased exercise, may help.

◆ Do not skip meals – eat little and often throughout the day.

◆ Healthy between-meal snacks are important if you want to gain weight.

◆ Make sure that at least 50–60% of your increased calories are in the form of complex carbohydrates (wholemeal bread, wholemeal pasta, brown rice, crispbread, cereal).

◆ Eat plenty of vegetables, including peas, beans and lentils.

◆ Eat plenty of fruit. Use as between-meal snacks, especially bananas.

◆ Try not to increase your fat intake to more than 30% of extra calories.

◆ Use semi-skimmed milk and low-fat dairy products so that weight gain does not come from eating fat.

◆ Exercise regularly, preferably for at least 30 minutes daily.

Note: If you are losing weight, or cannot gain it despite your best efforts, see your doctor.

FRESH PRODUCE
Although you will need to increase your food intake to gain weight, make sure your diet remains balanced. Eat as much fresh, simply prepared produce as possible.

CARBOHYDRATES
When trying to gain weight, at least half of your extra daily calories should be in the form of unrefined complex carbohydrates.

HEALTHY WEIGHT LOSS

Obesity is linked with premature death from a variety of common diseases.

It is just as important to look after your weight early in life as it is to prevent the onset of middle-age spread. Recent research shows that men who are prone to being overweight during their teen years are more than twice as likely to have a fatal heart attack by the age of 55, regardless of their adult weight.

One of the best ways to calculate the healthy weight range for your height is to work out your Body Mass Index (BMI). This is obtained by dividing your weight (in kilograms) by the square of your height (in metres):

$$BMI = \frac{Weight\ (kg)}{Height \times height\ (m^2)}$$

This calculation produces a number that can be interpreted by the coloured bands shown in the table below.

The BMI calculation is occasionally misleading. For example, trained body builders with excessive muscle mass may have a BMI of up to 30 kg/M^2 without having any excess fat on board.

For men, the healthy BMI range falls between 20 and 25, since this is not linked to an increased risk of weight-related deaths. Your risk of dying early in life doubles as your BMI rises from 30 to 40 kg/m^2.

The table (*opposite*) gives the weight range for men of different heights that correspond to a healthy BMI of 20–25. This lets you see at a glance whether or not you are in the healthy weight bracket. Remember that excess weight piles on when your food intake is greater than your energy output over a prolonged period of time.

LOSING WEIGHT SAFELY

The only way to lose weight is to eat fewer calories than you burn. The most successful way to do this is to lose only about 0.5–1 kg (1–2 lb) per week. If you try to lose weight more quickly, your health may suffer, and your body will fight you every step of the way since your metabolism will respond to a rapid decrease in food energy intake by becoming much more efficient.

Most experts now agree that to lose weight safely you need to:
◆ follow a low-fat diet
◆ exercise regularly in order to keep the weight off.
Because muscle tissue burns energy more rapidly than fat cells, increased

RATING YOUR WEIGHT

BMI (BODY MASS INDEX)	WEIGHT BAND
> 40	Dangerously obese
30–40	Obese
25–30	Overweight
20–25	Healthy
< 20	Underweight

muscle mass leads to an increased basal metabolic rate. The extra calories you eat after reaching your goal weight are, therefore, more likely to burn and less likely to stick if you follow an exercise programme. Weight training, for example, helps to build muscle mass and it also compensates for the natural loss of lean tissue that occurs as you grow older. Try attending an aerobics class regularly or take up cycling, swimming or jogging.

UNDERWEIGHT – are you eating enough?

HEALTHY – keep it there.

OVERWEIGHT – your health may suffer – do not get heavier.

OBESE – it is important that you lose weight.

DANGEROUSLY OBESE – treatment is urgently required.

GUIDELINES FOR BODY WEIGHT RELATIVE TO HEIGHT

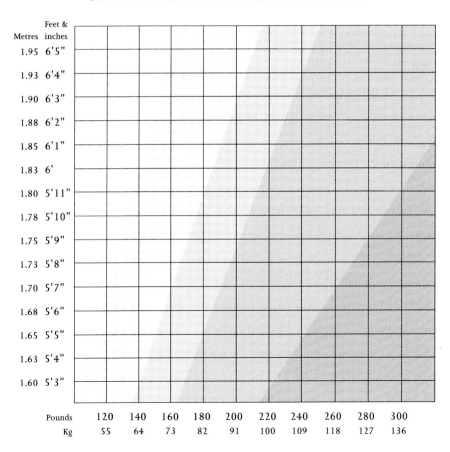

Metres	Feet & inches
1.95	6'5"
1.93	6'4"
1.90	6'3"
1.88	6'2"
1.85	6'1"
1.83	6'
1.80	5'11"
1.78	5'10"
1.75	5'9"
1.73	5'8"
1.70	5'7"
1.68	5'6"
1.65	5'5"
1.63	5'4"
1.60	5'3"

Pounds	120	140	160	180	200	220	240	260	280	300
Kg	55	64	73	82	91	100	109	118	127	136

STRATEGIES FOR WEIGHT LOSS

Aim to eat between 500 and 1,000 kcals per day less than you need to fuel your energy expenditure. But healthy weight loss also means looking at where your calories are coming from. For example, you should cut back on the amount of saturated (animal) fat you eat (*see pp. 38–41*). Instead of having red meat, go for lean meat such as chicken with the skin removed, and eat more fish and vegetarian meals (*see pp. 62–63*). Grill food rather than frying it and bake instead of roasting. If, as you ideally should, you are getting at least half your daily calories from complex carbohydrates, such as wholemeal bread, wholemeal pasta, cereals and baked potatoes, don't then smother them in calorific sauces or spreads.

Simple tips include:

◆ Switch to skimmed milk, which has almost 50 percent fewer calories per pint than whole milk. If you drink about 240 ml (half a pint) per day, you can save 450 calories a week.

◆ Use low-fat, low-calorie versions of all possible foods – such as vegetable spread, mayonnaise, yogurt, salad dressing, reduced-fat cheese, and reduced-fat monounsaturated spreads.

Red	**Green**	**Animal and dairy products**
Butter	Wholemeal bread	Semi-skimmed milk
Cream	Brown rice	Skimmed milk
Full cream milk	Unsweetened cereals	Cheese
Mayonnaise	Wholemeal pasta	Eggs (x 2 per week)
Oily salad dressings	Vegetables	Red meat
Salad cream	Fresh fruit	White meat
Fatty meat	Dried fruit	Cottage cheese
Fried foods	Unsweetened juice	Low-fat mayonnaise
Bacon	Seeds	Low-fat yogurt
Fatty sausages	Unsalted nuts	
Salami	Fish	
Paté		
Pastry		
Cream-based soups		
Sauces		
Chips		
Sugar		
Sweets		
Chocolate		
Cakes		
Biscuits		
Doughnuts		
Puddings		
Ice cream		
Sweetened cereals		
Jam, syrup		

CALORIE SOURCES
As a general rule, avoid foods on the red list, eat as much of the food on the green list as you like, and select frugally from the list of animal and dairy products.

EATING LESS

Ingrained eating habits are notoriously difficult to break. So, if you are trying to shed some weight, you may find some of the following tips useful in ringing the changes.

◆ Drink a large glass of sparkling mineral water before every meal – this will make you feel full more quickly so you end up eating less.

◆ If possible, try to eat the main meal of the day at lunchtime – your metabolic rate is higher during the day than it is in the evening, so calories are burned than are converted into fat. Try not to eat anything after 8 pm, since this is when your metabolism is sluggish.

◆ Always sit down at a table – do not eat while standing up. Sitting down to a meal encourages you to eat slowly; standing meals are associated with getting the food down your throat as quickly as possible.

◆ The advantage of eating slowly is that metabolic messages that you are feeling full start to come through before you have finished eating your food.

◆ Serve smaller portions of food than you think you need.

◆ If you feel that you are being deprived if your plate is not full, use a slightly smaller plate than usual.

◆ Eat more unrefined carbohydrates– these contain complex carbohydrates that trigger the release of serotonin, a chemical compound found in the in the brain that makes you feel fuller more quickly.

◆ Try to pause regularly while eating your food in order to slow the

BURNING EXTRA CALORIES

◆ Take every opportunity to walk rather than ride – and walk briskly rather than dawdling.

◆ Use the stairs instead of the lift. If you live on a high floor, start by walking up the last three or four flights of stairs. As you become fitter, start walking up the last five flights, and so on.

◆ Buy a bicycle (and safety equipment) or an exercise bike and use it regularly.

◆ If you don't have a dog, try to "borrow" one for daily walks. This may help to encourage you to exercise regularly. Jog every other minute to burn off extra calories.

◆ Swim as often as you can. There may be a pool near your work.

◆ For motivation, take up a team sport such as baseball or football.

mealtime down. Make an effort to put your knife and fork down while you chew your food.

◆ Concentrate on your food as you eat. Enjoy the tastes, textures and aromas of what you are eating. Do not read or watch TV at the same time, as you probably will just chew and swallow mechanically without really appreciating what you are eating. And, as a result, you will probably end up eating more.

◆ Use your imagination when substituting for high-fat ingredients. Do not assume that a low-fat alternative will not work. Yogurt, for example, is often a tasty substitute for cream.

◆ Keep a food diary and write down everything you eat – meals and snacks – if the scales refuse to budge after your best efforts.

AND FINALLY . . .

Eating fit means that you may never know just how much you needed it.

Your body will last you a lifetime – but just how long and how active that life will be is determined partly by what you eat.

Eating fit is one of the best ways to maintain your body so that it gives you long, trouble-free service. There is now little medical doubt that most diseases – some life-threatening and many life-shortening – have a dietary origin, although there remain many cases where this connection has not been fully understood.

Exciting new research shows that a healthy diet, providing plenty of fresh fruit and vegetables plus complex unrefined carbohydrates, will help you in a number of important ways, including:

◆ losing excess body fat
◆ maintaining a healthy weight
◆ obtaining all the vitamins, minerals and essential fatty acids you need for optimal health
◆ reducing your risk of coronary heart disease, high blood pressure, stroke, inflammatory diseases and some types of cancer.

Unless you are certain that your diet provides you with all the vitamins, minerals and essential fatty acids you need, why not consider taking a food supplement? Multinutrient supplements, containing sensible quantities of important micronutrients, provide an excellent safety net.

But no matter how important diet is, eating fit can only form part of your game plan for a long and healthy life.

You need to look at all aspects of your lifestyle and combine a healthy eating regime with regular exercise, a stress-relief programme and the sensible use of alcohol. Obviously, if you are a smoker, quitting is probably one of the most health-enhancing actions you can take in your life.

But taking care of your body does not mean that you cannot have a good time. In fact, eating fit should mean that the food you eat is tastier than ever before. If you eat organically grown fruit and vegetables and organically reared meat whenever you can, not only will you be doing your body some good, but you will have the added benefit of a fine-tasting meal.

Even if you do not have the time or the funds to go organic, seeking out quality produce, locally grown and seasonally available, and then cooking it in the most fat-free way will be a positive step along the road to a longer and healthier life. If cooking is not really your forte, get some simple cookbooks and experiment.

By eating a healthy diet you will find that you have more energy. If you have lost weight, you will find that it stays off; and feeling lighter will make you feel younger, better and more confident about yourself.

Diet, however, cannot cure everything, so don't become obsessed with calorie counting. Once you know the basic facts about food, then all you need is a little application and some common sense.

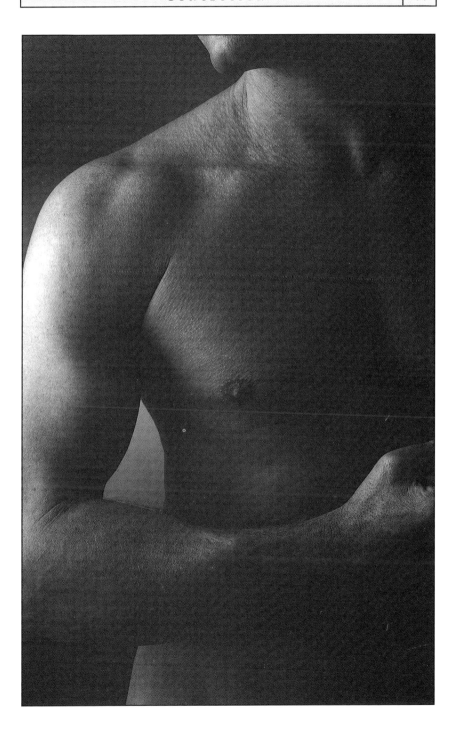

INDEX

Main mentions are in **bold** type.

Acknowledgments

Picture Credits

*All of the photographs in the book were taken by Laura Wickenden
except for the following:*
p.13 Dr. R. Clark and M. R. Goff/Science Photo Library
p.16 Richard Kirby, David Spears Ltd/Science Photo Library
p.17 Custom Medical Stock Photo/Science Photo Library
p.20 Secchi Lecaque/Rousell-Uclaf/CNRI/Science Photo Library;
BSIP, Secchi Lecaque/Science Photo Library
p.21 (top left) Robert Becker/Custom Medical Stock
Photo/Science Photo Library; (top right) Professor P. M. Motta
and S. Correr/Science Photo Library; (bottom) Professeur Luc
Montagnier, Institut Pasteur/CNRI/Science Photo Library
p.58 Superstock
Cover photography: Laura Wickenden
Illustrator: Mike Saunders p.25

The publishers also wish to thank:
Models: Jason, Brett Simmons, Sean
Stylist: Kendal Osbourn